"*Sometimes, trying to follow some of my reasoning is a little like trying to spoon ants.*"

Terry Goodkind
author of *Soul of Fire*

You may think this about several of the sections in this book. I'm not trying to be obtuse—this is just the way it comes out.

BRAIN-DAMAGE

A book about overcoming cognitive deficits
and creating the new you.

by

Dick Schmelzkopf

Edited by
Ellen Bennett & Denese Schmelzkopf

Emerald Ink Publishing
Houston, Texas

Copyright © 2001 Emerald Ink Publishing

All rights reserved. No part of this book may be reproduced or utilized in any form by any means, electronic or mechanical, including photocopying, recording or by any information or storage retrieval system, without permission in writing from the publisher, except printing or recording for the blind. Inquiries should be addressed to:
Emerald Ink Publishing, 16630 Imperial Valley Dr #149, Houston, TX 77060
E-mail: emerald@emeraldink.com.

Photo credits: Robert Palmer

Library of Congress
Cataloging of Publication Division
101 Independence Ave, S.E.
Washington, D. C. 20540-4320

Library of Congress Cataloging-in-Publication Data

Schmelzkopf, Richard Edward, 1939-
   Brain-damage with a cognitive deficit & pituitary dysfunction: a book about overcoming cognitive deficit and creating the new you / by Richard Edward Schmelzkopf
     p. cm.
Includes biographical references.
ISBN 1-885373- 35-X (alk. paper)
1. Schmelzkopf, Richard Edward, 1939---Health. 2. Pituitary gland--Tumors--Patients--United States--Biography. 3. Brain damage--Patients--United States--Biography. 4. Pituitary gland--Surgery--Patients-United States--Biography. I. Title.
RC280.P5 S35 2001
362.1'968'0092--dc21

Printed in the United States of America

ACKNOWLEDGEMENTS

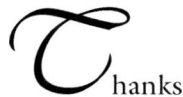hanks

I know all newly-published authors have thanks to give to a passel of people. This whole first chapter could be delegated to thanking people who have helped me or influenced me since my surgery. If I have left any key personnel out of this, please remember that I am brain-damaged, and that's no bull. This is the story of how it happened, to the best of my ability, to recall between phantom memory, poor memory and what people close to me have said. This is how I handled the changes in my life.

Denese, my wife, known to friends and relatives as Denny, is an incredible woman. The statistics for mates staying with brain-damaged significant others are horrendous: about seventy-five percent of the mates leave. They just can't live with the other person having a nick out of the gray matter. Not only has she stuck around, but she has also become the sole bread winner and is keeping me in the manner to which I have become accustomed, and then some. She has developed the attitude that we will win, no matter what the rest of the world is doing. Through these last few years she has lived with my inadequacies and mood swings that would put Hollywood to shame. She has put up with my different egos getting in the way, some of them being sexual, male, and head-of-the-house. Life's ride for the last few years has been a monster roller coaster excursion. She was able to hang on through the stratospheric highs, the Mariana trench lows, life's loop-de-loops, and the ever-present phantom memories. I would add to this my very selective memory, as I have no choice what is remembered, be it important or not. That's just to name a few of the obstacles she has had to overcome to give me love and support.

My in-laws, George and Sara Nell, get a big hand. They keep inviting me to family events even though I may drool a little in public and make an embarrassing moment or two. They must still love me—they have a couple of entries in my dragon collection and I know I wouldn't send dragons to someone I didn't care for.

My family, Mother, Sue, and Phil, and their families keep sending love, and make sure I realize there is no pressure on me from them. And to Howie, recently deceased, for taking care of my mother those years. It was a relief for me to know she was in good, loving hands.

If it weren't for Dr. Guida Jackson and her graduate students who were kind enough to let me join their critique groups, you wouldn't be reading this. My thanks and encouragement to our tiny critique group, Jim Eric and of course Blood and Guts Mel (even though it took easily twice the time to go through my stuff). I must quote Guida here: "If you are a writer... write."

Those words of encouragement have sent me to this computer more times than I can count.

Project ReEntry, my rehab shop, all of the Angels (counselors) and staff have helped me find my weak areas and bolster them up, as well as help me create the new Dick Schmelzkopf. Along with the angels I must thank my fellow rehabbers for the encouragement they have given me. Special thanks to Dr. Larry Pollock and Russ Shanks for their support and encouragement through this period. Although these two guys run the place, they always had time to listen to me and be a sounding board. Other rehabbers and Angels will be mentioned throughout this book.

Marta, the chief brain-peeker (psychologist), always helped me see a way to overcome a negative thought; it is all a matter of how you want to look at a problem. Essentially, she used to say, "Fix it or fight it." It is so much easier to fix it, especially with her help.

Thanks to all the guys and gals along the way who helped me get my doctorate in survival—there is another book on all the ways I have been helped.

To the guys at Steve's Rock and Poker Parlor who taught me the value and cost of paying attention to what is going on this minute (and if I'm playing low spade in the hole I won't get out if I have the deuce of spades down) and for belly laughs too numerous to count, a special thank you. As anybody in the rehab business will tell you, there is no greater therapy than a good solid belly laugh.

The Spring Creek Dart Association never once threw a dart at me for being a slow math person. They knew that my internal calculator had a serious flaw and I appreciate their understanding.

Thanks to the Supper Club for helping me with my social skills and etiquette, even though I have committed enough faux pas to be a life-long member.

Thank you, Bob Knight for sticking with me on the pool game and getting me going with the basics again, and putting up with my fits of temper because I couldn't do it like I used to.

Guida Jackson recommended that I call Chris because he specializes in books about people overcoming personal adversity. When I sat down with Chris he told me "Guida's connection opened the door for you. If you have a good story I'll look at it." Chris Carson at Emerald Ink Publishing convinced me that I have a story to tell that can help folks. Thanks for taking a flier on an unknown writer, Chris. I hope together we can make a buck or two and help some folks.

Thanks to the bridge group for showing me the value of good communications while playing this game. Seven no-trump, doubled and re-doubled can be challenging. They taught me the value of counting to thirteen and tracking trump.

Thank you Texas for giving me a top shelf living for all those good years, then helping me when I was down and out.

A Word from the Spouse

When I was a teenager, I saw this motto carved on a tombstone: ECCE HOMO. It piqued my curiosity and I looked it up in the dictionary. It means, "Behold, A Man." The words brought visions of knights in shinning armor and crusaders fighting for righteousness. I thought it would be the highest accolade you could give someone for leading an exemplary life. I hoped that someday I would have someone in my life who would live up to this lofty expectation.

The book you are going to read is about such a man.

I didn't realize until after Dick's surgery how special he was. It wasn't because I realized how short life is and how lucky I was to still have him. It was because I learned each day of his rehabilitation that he was now like everyone else. Sounds strange, doesn't it?

I didn't know that men had challenges communicating with women. I didn't know they were reluctant to discuss their personal feelings. It was hidden from me that they were not prone to do sweet, sentimental things. I never gave thought to how soft and yet so strong they could be. None of these things came to mind until after the doctors removed part of my husband's brain.

He woke in ICU and I thought a miracle had happened. He was still here. He was still Dick. It would take me several years to realize a different person was residing in his body. Several years of watching him fight and claw, inching back to whom he used to be.

Had he started out being like everyone else, he wouldn't be where he is today. Today, I see a man who through sheer force of character has overcome some of the most difficult challenges a human can face. Not just challenges of body, but challenges of mind. Challenges that don't show; outwardly at least. Challenges no one else sees. Challenges that might have overcome everything he means to me.

It's been over six years since that day in ICU. I wish I could tell you everything is back the way it used to be, but I can't. Nothing will ever be the same. What I can tell you, though, is that Dick has emerged on the other side of recovery with a strength of will that would make even the most unbelieving say *Ecce Homo*. And I love him still.

Denese Schmelzkopf

FROM THE SURGEON

*D*ear Mr. Schmelzkopf,

I read with great interest your synopsis; the amount of knowledge that the public has of problems like yours is minimal; education in that regard is badly needed.

The number of people with cognitive deficit, as you are aware, is quite large. The understanding of the causes remains limited. Only people with determination and willpower as big as yours (and who have the fortune of having as beautiful and cooperative a person as your wife at their side) can, with the assistance of expert Rehabilitation teams, make inroads and in the process create "the new me."

Thank you for allowing me to make these comments.

Raul Sepulveda, M.D.
Dick's Surgeon

INTRODUCTION

The publication of this book by Dick Schmelzkopf gives me great pleasure, because the first time I met him, I wouldn't have made a very large bet on its ever happening. I first encountered Dick several years ago in a creative writing class I taught at Montgomery College. From the beginning, he distinguished himself as being different. Most of the other students were working on contemporary adult novels. Dick was writing a fanciful story about a benign wizard and an amethyst-eyed dragon named Purpose. It was through the very first chapter of his story that I saw two elements of Dick's character that would serve him in good stead: his imagination and his sense of humor. Although his story was fresh, imaginative, and peppered with bits of wisdom and insight, the fundamental mechanics of writing were sorely lacking. It was many weeks before I learned the reason for Dick's "handicap," weeks during which he worked many times harder than the other students, meticulously rewriting each chapter according to my notes and corrections. This gave me a sense of three more of his traits: his determination, tenacity, and especially his enthusiasm, which never flagged, no matter how many errors he had to correct. It was not until I learned the nature of the obstacles he had already overcome before arriving at that point did I have an inkling of the heart of the man and the courage. Dick's writing continued to show significant improvement over the months and years that followed. Early in his new career, he was asked to make a tape for other people undergoing similar physical rehabilitation. This was his first publishing success, and the whole class celebrated with him. Eventually he got his own website, where visitors could read about the adventures of the wizard and the dragon named Purpose. The recounting for this current book of the miraculous but tediously long transformation following his devastating brain debilitation must have been a wrenching, painful chore for Dick. To face the horrors once would be difficult enough; to go back in memory and re-live them in order to share the story takes an uncommon degree of valor. Ultimately, the success of a story depends upon how much empathy the reader feels for the main character, the "hero" in this case, the author. The traits that I have enumerated here, imagination, a sense of humor, determination, enthusiasm, tenacity, heart, courage, honesty, candor, uncommon valor, describe a true hero. They are the stuff of which epics are made. I can hardly wait to read this book myself.

Guida Jackson
Dick's Writing Guru

Contents

A Look Back 1
Flashback to Disaster Super Nova Headache 5
At the Emergency Center 7
Surgery 9
Intensive Care Unit 11
Quality of Life 15
What Does Brain-Damaged Mean? 17
Flooding 21
Peace of Mind 25
Religion 29
Fetish 31
Naps 35
Lids, Caps, Stoppers and Tops 37
Chocolate Freak 39
Beard Power 41
Heroes 43
Airport Flooding 45
Working with My Hands 47
Anger 49
Anger: A History 51
I'm Really Smokin' Now 53
A Tool to Use, A Strategy 65
A Broken Recognizer 69
Instant Gratification 71
Convalescing at Home 73
Multi-Tasking 77
Pets 79

Grief 83
Mining for Kitty-Gold 85
Patience & Frustration 87
Vocabulary 93
Books 95
Texan 97
Dr. See & TRC 99
Medications 101
Dr. Z, Endocrinologist 103
Education 105
Testing 107
Test Results 109
Angels at Rehab 113
First Day at Project Re-entry 115
Day to Day Rehab 119
I Finally Stopped Drooling in Public or
I Know Who I Used to Be, But Who Am I Now? 125
Who's Brain-Damaged? 127
Awareness & Beauty 129
A Writer 131
Bourbon 135
Add Wonderment to Brain-damaged 139
Cecil B. DeMille? or Steven Spielberg? 141
Creativity 145
Reading To Learn 147
Negativity, The Terrible Twos & The Rebellious Teens 149
Flooding While Dressing 151
Frustration 153
Sometimes It Just Doesn't Go Right 155

Those Who Stick With You 159
Pool 161
Pool and Darts 163
Flexibility, Panic, Communications 165
Poker 167
Party Bridge 173
Supper Club 175
Silliness 177
The Upside To Being Brain-Damaged 179
Emotions Run Wild 181
Internal Thermostat 183
To You, For You, The Reader 185
Afterword From His Counselor 187
From The Director of the Facility 193

A Look Back

As my wife and I stroll along this Caribbean beach, all I can think of is what a roller coaster ride these last few years have been. We have been married for thirty years, loving it, and loving each other. I get a multitude of flashbacks going through my mind at one time. The first flashback is how rosy our world was before all these challenging things happened to me. I should say us, because it sure has had an impact on my wife's life as well as mine. She went from co-breadwinner to the only breadwinner. Not exactly what I had promised her when we got married. I used to kid her and say, "I'll have you wearing diamonds as big as horse apples."

Now she tells me, "Not to worry—diamonds are too ostentatious to wear on the beach anyway."

God I love that woman!

Before moving to Houston, I was a lobbyist and National Government Sales Manager for a large manufacturing company. Washington DC, the Hill, was my beat. That was a fun period. I did lots of entertaining at all levels. This is where Denny and I first got together.

We moved to Houston during the boom years and sold high-tech, high-priced electronic equipment to the petrochemical and public utilities worlds. My wife and I worked as a team through many years and several companies. We sold the 'man-machine' interface for process control, energy management systems and supervisory control and data acquisition systems, as well as multi-media learning work stations and performance support systems. We had what is known as a satellite office. The company's main office might be in Pennsylvania or Wisconsin, but we had our local office in our home. At different times we were responsible for anything from a five-state area around Texas to the whole United States.

We were pretty much in charge of our own time and schedules. So when we got ahead of our quota we might plan a long weekend in Cancun. As long as our sales numbers were up and the customers were happy, the company didn't care how we ran our territory. So we worked extra hard because we liked those long weekends in the Caribbean. It was not unusual to start very early in the morning to work the phone with the East Coast and work late at night with the West Coast. We thrived on long hours. We worked very well together and enjoyed it. I can safely say we worked together as effortlessly as teeth and tongue. Few husbands and wives can work together, much less from sunrise to sunset day after day. But we loved it. It seemed to make our love for each other grow, and our communications improve. After fifteen years or so, my wife decided she wanted to get involved with something that didn't have the technology changing weekly, like computers have a propensity to do.

Not too long after that my work started to pale and I was fired from my job. I am told now that the tumor probably had something to do with the change in my ability to produce. I had been making a good deal of money for several years. We had a great stock portfolio and several rental properties. We would fly to the Caribbean every couple of months. Life was good. Our net worth was in seven figures, most everyone's family dreams. I wasn't worried at all about getting another job; I had an excellent name in the industry as a top-notch sales person. After a couple of years of interviews and still no job offer that I was interested in, my wife was providing the sole support. Meanwhile, we were living at the same level as before. All this time we were depleting our investments, thinking I would be working soon.

I remember thinking how unfortunate: just when you think you have the world in your pocket, you can lose it all. I remember feeling badly for my wife. After all, I promised her the good life, and we were losing it. I didn't think things could get any worse. Then it happened.

FLASHBACK TO DISASTER
SUPER NOVA HEADACHE

One Sunday we were sitting around the house not doing anything special, just reading the paper and doing the crossword puzzle together, which is our customary Sunday. I got a monster headache. I thought it was sinus problems. My wife drove me to one of those little quickie clinic places. The doctor said he also thought it was a sinus problem. After all, living in Houston, it is not unusual to blame anything from athlete's foot to dandruff on allergies or sinus problems. Or for that matter, just any old ache or pain. He gave me some pain pills and said if I got double vision to go to an emergency room immediately. Sure enough three hours later I looked up at the clock in our living room and I saw two clocks. Even with the pills, the pain was excruciating. My headache was a super nova.

AT THE EMERGENCY CENTER

At that point Denny and I were scared; I mean really scared. I was actually shaking. My wife said I was shaking like a cocker spaniel passing a peach seed. (I've never seen a dog pass a peach seed, but I can imagine how scared the little pooch would be. Just like the cocker, I had no idea what the pain was all about.)

We went to the emergency room at N. W. Medical Center. There were numerous tests, MRI, CAT Scan, and the full battery of biological and physical testing—you know the type of thing I'm talking about: "Squeeze my hand, now look up here, now look over there, can you feel this? Does your family have a history of any of this, or any of that?" (I was adopted, so I couldn't give them any historical medical data. That always seems to frustrate the doctors, although it doesn't bother me at all.) Blood and urine tests, pressure checks, temperature and other unnamed electronics had the doctors and nurses running. Everything was going well for me, but the look on the faces of the professionals was not encouraging.

SURGERY

*B*etween my wife and me, I refer to "BS" as *before surgery* and "AS," as *after surgery*. This designation helps me establish time lines when we are discussing memory or events.

The doctor came back and told us I had a tumor on my pituitary gland that had ruptured and was putting pressure on my optic nerve. I could go blind or even die.

They said they must do *emergency brain surgery now*! Fortunately for me, Dr. Raul Sepulveda was on call. Thank the powers that be! I might also add, much to the chagrin of the insurance company, he was not on the insurance company's list of recommended surgeons. (This shows what *they* know. We would pay dearly for this in time, effort and money.)

The pituitary gland is located just about the center of the head. Dr. Sepulveda and his team could not use the safer method of going up through the sinus cavity, they would need to go through my skull, and that meant twelve hours of emergency surgery. The surgeon would have to disturb the gray matter of the frontal lobe to get to the tumor and this would result in some type of brain trauma. The doctor assured me that without this operation I would go blind, there was no doubt about it. The repercussions from going in through the side of the skull and disturbing the frontal lobe could vary tremendously. There was no sure way to know the extent of the damage until the operation was over. The problems could be many - they gave me a laundry list of possibilities ranging from partial or total blindness to a loss of cognitive capabilities, which could include a loss of any number of functions. Or, I might come out of the operation a blithering idiot. The list went on and on. I was then *officially* shaking in my boots; Denny wasn't much cooler, so she tells me.

    I cannot tell this story without interjecting some humor. Humor is one of the things I lost after the operation: I didn't laugh for two years. Now I take great joy in looking at this whole thing and picking out the humorous aspects. From time to time I will share some ironies, strange goings-on, unusual events, and lessons learned. The first lesson would be: *Don't have emergency brain surgery without checking with your insurance company.* (I say this with tongue in cheek. You would think the term emergency brain surgery would connote: operate now!) Even with all the trouble I had because Dr. Sepulveda was not on their list I wouldn't trade him for a covey of other surgeons.

    As it turned out, Dr. Sepulveda was not able to remove the entire tumor. He had to leave about ten percent, with a caveat that this thing could grow back, so I will indulge in the great sport of having an MRI every six to twelve months for the rest of my days. When I do, I have learned to put any claustrophobic feelings aside and bring out my meditation skills. The MRIs are a minor inconvenience when you consider the alternative.

INTENSIVE CARE UNIT

After the twelve hours of emergency surgery, they placed me in intensive care. My stay there stretched to twelve days. My surgeon assured me it was a picture-perfect operation. Besides not becoming a vegetable, I would have absolutely no scar, so it wouldn't be mistaken for a botched job by Dr. Frankenstein. Dr. Sepulveda tells me he lectures throughout the world using my operation as a case study on how to do it right. I told him I would be willing to go with him to the more interesting places, like any of the Caribbean islands. I could just sit in a chair on the stage and he could point at me. I told him I wouldn't drool too much, but he wouldn't go for it.

I know of other cases where the patients didn't fare so well; they ended up with serious brain damage. I ended up with a non-functioning pituitary gland, and I still have a small piece of tumor in my head that could grow back at any time. (I didn't want to hear that, but as time goes on there are a lot of things I don't want to hear. I have the attitude that I want them to tell me the way it is, not the way I want it to be.) The lack of a pituitary gland lends some additional complications to the post surgical diagnosis, recovery, and the rest of my life.

During the period I spent in intensive care all flavors of specialists came to see me trying to evaluate and determine just what I had lost. The greatest loss seems to be in the executive functioning areas. This includes a plethora of problems. Again, the laundry list is long, extensive and convoluted. A little like a catch twenty-two: you know if you lose this, it affects this area over here and when you don't have that, it means you can't do this other thing. When I go to rehabilitation I find out how all these things play together, or maybe I should say, don't play together. I will give you a blow-by-blow of these wonderments as I go along. The losses affected long- and short-term memory. This reminds me of a quote my wife read to me from Readers Digest, "My memory is the thing I forget with." There is lots of that going on and a lot more to come. I didn't realize it then, but I was going to have to get used to not remembering things. To this day my memory is very selective and I have absolutely no choice of what it remembers and what it doesn't. I phrased that as though my memory were a separate entity. That's because most of the time that is the way my memory interacts with the rest of my mind. These losses also influenced implementation of procedures and problem solving skills: try starting your car, cooking, shopping or working with your computer if you can't remember procedures. The things I gained are attributes that I would just as soon do without. For instance, I now have cognitive inflexibility, all the better for not being able to have an open mind. Some of the other all-time favorites that I acquired are maximum frustration and major depression. These two play well together. A little like Abbott and Costello doing "Who's On First Base?" If you think the little fat guy got frustrated and angry, hang in there. Let's see if you can empathize with us cognitively challenged folks. I will get frustrated, then the frustration will feed the depression, all because I can't do something or work something out. Or how about being in a general depression, then try to get myself out of it and getting so frustrated I would like to scream, "God, why me?" Then let's throw in impulsivity and poor visual scanning. As I said, all of these problems cascade to affect many other areas. With the pituitary dysfunction comes constant tiredness and sexual dysfunction. Being in the hospital, the sexual problem didn't mean much yet. But after being home awhile, all of these problems would become devastating. Having had a very active sexual life with my wife, this added to the frustration, the pressure I put on myself, and the depression. Merely hearing about the sex thing from the doctor was bad enough, experiencing it brought this whole fiasco to a new level. I felt I wasn't a whole man. The sexual dysfunction would become a worm in my brain, eating away, leaving in its wake huge piles of waste that would turn into depression, guilt and fear.

    I am very fortunate that the head nurse of the ICU, Priscilla, is a friend of the family. I knew I would receive the best of care, not only I, but the whole ICU area. At first I felt very uncomfortable getting sponge baths from the nurses, be it male or female. In the end I was very grateful for the time they spent with me either keeping my body clean or my spirits up. ICU nurses have a tough row to hoe and I'm mighty thankful for the care I received. Especially the cold soft drinks they would bring me; I had a thirst that could not be quenched, like pouring water on the Sahara. I appreciate the visits from the supper-club folks, even though I wasn't always aware of what was going on.

I remember Donna, (she's a long tall Texan) bringing me big Texas smiles and saying to us, "Howdy, how ya'll doin?"—this with a Texas drawl that would put a smile on even a curmudgeon's face. Sure does make ICU a warmer place.

QUALITY OF LIFE

*Q**uality of life* means different things to different people. When I initially got out of surgery, the first cogent thought I had was, "I could be taken out of this world at any moment for any reason. I am mortal and there will be an end. As of this minute I am going to enjoy life more, do more of the things that I have always wanted to do. I am going to love more, live more, do more, and help more."

To quote Tom Wolfe when he got out of the hospital after a serious heart operation:

"Count the days you have left."

Whatever life I have left will be lived with *my idea of* "quality of life."

A great song says:
"I'm going to live till I die."

Me too! Let me add to that, a line from a Sammy Davis Jr. song:
"I want to live, not merely survive."

WHAT DOES BRAIN-DAMAGED MEAN?

*I*t is relatively easy to spot a handicapped person if they are an amputee. How do you spot a person who is handicapped because they are cognitively challenged?

I tend to tell people up-front that I am brain-damaged, not all of the time, but mostly. I like to do this before I make a mistake of some sort, because I would rather have them know I am brain-damaged than think I was stupid.

When people are talking down to me, or leaning towards baby talk, or how you might talk to a favorite pet, I say to them, "Hey, I had a little brain damage; they didn't give me a lobotomy." It is a hard way to bring them to reality but the shock of the statement generally will bring the conversation around to where we are all on the same level. Does it mean we're slow, stupid, dumb, an idiot, incapable, retarded, challenged, half-witted or maybe mentally ill? Some folks who don't know us might even say insane. People who do know us will say, "Not insane, but maybe a little crazy. If not crazy, certainly a carrier," because at times we drive those around us a little crazy.

Here are some more *are we's*. This is a good one: *hebetudinous*, which means the state of being dull. In some areas I am, maybe. As a rule I would say no. (Not that I'm biased, mind you.) Idiot? Roget's Thesaurus says, "One deficient in judgment and good sense." Somewhat, I suppose I can say the same for most of the people I know. Everyone has shown poor judgment at one time or another. This amounts to, "Has every decision you have ever made been the right one?" Probably not, but you may want to check on your life and death decisions. I don't handle the money in our family and there is a good reason for that: my wife makes better money decisions than I do. As a matter of fact, she did BS (Before Surgery) as well. I don't want to know from money. It's frustrating just thinking about it. However, I've made better poker decisions than she does and for some reason, I still do.

Retarded? "Having a limited ability to learn and understand." Some, yes. But then again, I'm learning to be a writer. I'm learning new words, I'm learning how to intertwine plots, subplots and characters: I'm learning plot care and feeding. I'm learning how to overcome cognitive deficits, and I'm doing it on a daily basis. A little slower than your average bear, but I'm nipping away at it as are my fellow rehabbers who are serious about creating the new person. How many people do you know who are learning new things on a daily basis and using them? For us, it is a matter of survival in a world that considers us less, slower, and so on. Does this seem to look like a glass ceiling, ladies? Now if you're black, short, one-eyed, Jewish and have a speech impediment, you may have it a little tougher. Sammy made it; we can too. Brain-damaged means we may be a little slower in some areas, but don't count us out. Remember the tortoise and the hare.

The next thing you know one of us will be writing a book like Dr. Claudia L. Osborn's, "Over my Head" or taking some other leading characterization in life. She certainly is a role model for me. Brain- damaged means you should take another look at the person. What are their strengths? Does this person have any areas that I may be able to help and support? What assets does this person bring to the table? Are they conscientious? Are they honest? Can I count on them? Are they communicating? Are they willing to learn? How do they handle new things? To most of us cognitively-challenged folks everything is new because we're looking at things with different eyes. New things may be tough, but we get a lot of practice at it.

You know what they say, "How do you get to Carnegie Hall?"

"Practice."

We get a lot of practice on new things. Give us a chance to be your friend, lover, or employee, maybe even sounding board. I guarantee you will see a different slant on most subjects that you might discuss. I will be a prolific, proficient, interesting writer and story teller. Take that to the bank.

FLOODING

I believe it is impossible for someone to understand flooding, unless you flood. I make reference to it all through this book. Imagine the worst worrier, hypochondriac, anal-retentive person you have ever known and suddenly, through the miracle of brain surgery, you have become that person. You have no choice what pops into your head and you cannot choose what you will think about a particular problem or situation. The thoughts, however bizarre, are there and seem to have slipped into your mind.

It is similar to *selective memory* combined with *phantom memory*. You have no choice what is remembered, any more than having a particular memory that is vivid, and finding out that it never took place and you have no history that you can rely on to build a defense. You may have only vague memory anyway. That's a nice start; now add that you are claustrophobic, are dumped into a coffin with a dead guy, and then dropped into a cave where no one will ever find you. The incoming data is fast and furious. It doesn't make any difference if the input is life-threatening or a matter of 'I'll stop and get milk on the way home.'

You would think that a guy who has trouble with any kind of multi-tasking wouldn't be able to have several thoughts at the same time. Not true. It is all flood material, although I must say that the heavier the matter, the bigger the rush, confusion, indecision and pressure. But, I repeat, incoming flooding can come from anywhere. I see something, or remember something, or somebody says something to me. It is imperative that I help you, the reader, understand what flooding is to the cognitively-impaired person. When I get a bad one it can blow me away for hours. I become non-communicative, withdrawn, depressed, sorry for myself, mad at myself, mad at God, but mostly mad at myself for letting the little things get to me, even though I have no choice in the matter.

I have had several bad *floodings*. Let me share some of the beauties with you. To simulate a flooding, read this next part very fast:

> Ruby, my nineteen-eighty-four red Cadillac convertible, is a pride and joy. Over the weekend I couldn't get it started. Should I finally trade it in? Am I putting too much money into it? Didn't I just have the whole electrical system replaced? Should I call AAA? Should I call my mechanic, in whom I have infinite faith? I tried jump starting it myself. That didn't work. As I was going to make the call to AAA someone came to the door. The dogs started barking. (Denny was in her office trying to work. It was my job to keep the dogs quiet.) If I brought them into my office then I couldn't hear. We had had termite damage and the man who was going to fix it was a friend of Dino's, one of my poker buddies. Would this guy give me a fair deal on repairs? I hadn't heard a thing from the other guy I wanted to bid the job—should I wait? Should I have called Sears for a third bid? Denny was to leave on a two day business trip. Could I handle all the stuff she does when she is home? I couldn't get Shardak to take his medication;

I'd tried cheese, peanut butter, and yogurt. He would eat the good stuff and spit out the pills. Bob was coming over to shoot pool. I hate it when I shoot poorly, and I know it is no fun for Bob. I should practice before he gets here. I almost forgot I would have darts tomorrow. I should practice darts as well. I didn't want to let my teammates down. I moved the cats from Denny's office to the spare bedroom beside my office. Would they be able to find the food and litter box okay? I wanted to try that new kitty litter that looks like plastic. Our big dog Shardak is twelve now and he suffers greatly from arthritis and can't make it out to relieve himself. I have wrapped a belt around his stomach just in front of his back legs, to help him up and help move him to wherever Denny and I happen to be. He enjoys being in my office with me, so that is kind of a starting place. I know I'm going to have to put him down soon. My heart is heavy with that thought. I love the beast like a brother or a son; he is a best friend. He gives me unquestioned love, nuzzles me on bad days, comes to me when I'm emotionally down, which has been so often these last few years. Denny has one more homeopathic medicine she wants to try. Wouldn't it be great if we could have him around for another couple of years with quality of life? That is a must! Greg called from National, my car place. I need a transmission overhaul. I'm sure these guys wouldn't rip me off. Ruby is a beauty but...."Fix her," I told him. The other termite guy called. I liked Dino's friend better. Denny said to call and give him the job. I've got to return that stuff to the drug store; it didn't work. I've got to remember to clean the house while Denny is in Dallas. That bird feeder fell down; I'll fix that when I blow off the porch. I wonder why we're not getting any hummingbirds this year. It is time, isn't it? I'll have to call the Audubon Society and check on it. Didn't I just put new hummingbird food out? I wonder if it is okay. Denny is going to take me to Mexico for a couple of days, a new place that should be fun. What do I want to take?

If you read that really fast, and as you are absorbing the first outpour, you answer the second while you're thinking about the third to answer before the fourth, then you may get the feel for how jumbled my mind gets.

I haven't yet worked out a method to keep this phenomenon called flooding from starting. If I find the answer and can bottle it, we will have a much better world. I believe folks who aren't brain-damaged go through this in a less threatening way. As best I can recall, I did B.S. (Before Surgery), though nothing this extreme. Regular people experience a lot of the things that cognitively-challenged people do; it's just that our episodes are much deeper, more traumatic, more frequent, wilder, longer—well, you get the idea. I am told this by people who are supposed to know, and I have faith in their wisdom. In a word, flooding is one of my worst things.

PEACE OF MIND

When someone asks, "What kind of car do you drive?" I give them the full pedigree. I have a 1984 Cadillac Eldorado Biarritz, limited edition, ruby red convertible that I call Ruby. My wife says "There is a lot of your personality tied up in this car."

Maybe so. I like the car. It is fun to drive. With the top up, it is just another car, but with the top down, it makes me feel like a million dollars. When I drive by a group of younger folks, I usually get a thumbs up from the group. The point I want to make is that when Ruby gets a cold or doesn't act properly, I have a place to take her where I know they will treat her and me right.

I know these guys will not rip me off. Bruce, Greg and their team of mechanics at National Transmission understand how important this car is to me. They treat the car like it was their own. As a matter of fact, Greg had owned a Caddy just like mine, when I first started going to these guys. From a user's point of view, I figure Greg's knowledge gives them an inside track.

Get electricians, plumbers, handymen, lawncare folks, doctors and lawyers you can trust. Our CPA, Terry, is not only looking out for our interests, he is also a very nice guy with a nice new bride. At the Tea Room, there are special people, Margaret and the rest of the Tea Room Gang. When she found out I was going to be published, she volunteered The Tea Room for a book signing lunch.

Our vet, Dr. Bill Drow, and his gang of ever-helpful saints have helped us through many a tight spot with our beasties over the past twenty years.

I want to get to know people; I want them to know me. Whoever you must deal with, tell them your situation. If you're brain-damaged, let them know. Most people want to help. I get a lot of "My, you don't look brain-damaged...Aahh, I mean." I've got to jump in and bail them out, so they don't get super uncomfortable. The first thing I say is, "I understand," then go about giving them as much education as they will allow me to on the subject of brain-damage/cognitive-rehabilitation.

Mike, at Molly's, the pub where I play darts, and all the gals who deliver beer to me during darts realize that something is not quite right, but I think they believe it is insanity and not brain-damage. Mike was my dart hero when I first started playing. Now, thanks to him and some other *"A" flite darters*, I look at him as a competitor. Mind you, I'm still not near Mike's level, but I don't think he walks on water anymore.

These people would never dream of letting me get into trouble—any kind of trouble. I trust them. We have good relationships.

Charlie, our local handyman, is a sweetheart. He is retired oil-patch trash. I say that lovingly. I can't count the things around our house that he has set right. He does a good solid job for an honest dollar.

All of the people I have mentioned are examples of people who know my situation and do everything they can to make life true and honest in their dealings with me. If any tradesmen or professionals were to take advantage of an impaired individual, the courts would look at that violation of trust very seriously. I don't believe the violator would ever take advantage of that type of situation again. If it happens to you and you don't want to take them to court, remember this old street saying. "Do me bad once, shame on you; do me bad twice, shame on me." We cognitively-challenged folks have enough to worry about. Get peace of mind where you can. There are honest tradesmen and professionals out there. Find them, and reward them by telling your friends and neighbors.

RELIGION

I haven't had one friend come to me with a T-shirt that says, "The streets really are paved with gold." Nor have I seen a baseball cap that says, "Pearly Gates Bar & Grill." I've seen no postcards or pictures of angels floating on clouds playing harps. So who is to say what heaven really is? My idea of heaven is just as possible as the next guy's.

    I don't believe in any particular religion. I was baptized and confirmed a Lutheran. I almost married a Catholic girl, so I went through their conversion material. My first serious encounter was Jewish; her father enjoyed the religion and tried to inform me. Denny majored in religion at one of the universities. She and I have had an interest in religion in one way, shape or form since our marriage. So after dabbling in it for some forty years, the one thing that I have decided is that none of the formal, organized religions agree on much. I surmised that if this is the case there is absolutely no reason why I couldn't form my own beliefs, and I have. If someone asks me if I am a religious person I tell them no, but I am a spiritual person. I talk to God as I talk to anybody else. There are no 'thees' and 'thous' and that jazz. When I see a beautiful bird, day, or what have you, I tell God, "God, you did a good job on hummingbirds" or "Thanks for another beautiful Texas day."

When I think about the poor soul who believes that his God does not allow pets in heaven, it only confirms that my God is a much better God than his. The bull about pets not having souls so they can't get past the pearly gates is just that: bull. Who says what constitutes a soul? If you knew Shardak, you might question your basic premise and your God. In my heaven if you have been a good soul and tried to do the right thing (and that includes kindness to pets) when Saint Peter opens those gates, Gabriel blows his horn. It doesn't make any difference if you were a good dog or a good person, you're in.

My thoughts on religion and God haven't changed much from BS (Before Surgery) to AS (After Surgery) except to add Quality of Life. This has a lot more meaning now than it did BS. If you believe in a higher power, remember: that power seems to have a mind of Its/Her/His own. That power could take you any time it wants. But, so do *you* have a mind. Add *quality of life* to your personal credo. Don't be the person who says, "I wish I had done so and so." If it is important to you, do it!

FETISH

I have developed a fetish or two. This means that there are things that I just *must* do. As an example, I wouldn't consider going out of the house without shining my boots first. I believe this is a good fetish. Because my internal thermostat doesn't work worth a darn, I now always wear a sport coat when I leave the house. The temperature in Houston is mostly warm to hot. The buildings in Houston are mostly cold as a well-digger's belt buckle, so I wear a sport coat. I can always take it off if it gets too warm. I find I mostly wear the coat. It makes no difference to me if it is a formal occasion or casual, a coat is part of the "uniform of the day." Now this can pose a problem. When I want to look particularly well dressed, I try to match my shirt to my coat and trousers. Many a time I have changed clothes several times to try and get a better match. My wife says that I have extra interest in my appearance now because of the year I spent running around in nothing but snuggie-suits (sweat suits). I tell her, "I believe I take extra care about dressing because I wouldn't want people to think you were hanging around with some guy that dressed like a slob."

After all, I will be judged by the people I am seen with. If my wife is seen hanging around with a jerk, then my wife would be perceived as not caring. I wouldn't want people to think that I am running around with a non-caring person. Would you? If this makes sense to you, you probably need to come with me on Tuesdays and Thursdays to rehab!

My wife is very organized. We keep a list on the side of the refrigerator of the things we need to buy at the next shopping expedition. There are certain things that we keep backups of. We have been doing this for a long time, so it's not like a new thing. A few things we keep backed up are toilet paper, paper towels, milk, small and large Zip-lock Bags and toothpaste. I'm sure most houses have this same type of system. However, I have added to this backup supply list something fierce: I now have backup underwear and socks. I get terribly mad at myself if I let any thing slip and don't put it on the list. It is standard practice in our house if you use the next to the last one of these items it goes immediately on the grocery list. Fortunately, my wife puts up with these little quirks. If I get too involved with the little things, she reminds me that they are not life and death actions or items. This statement tends to bring me back to reality. After all, how serious can it be to run out of milk when the store is only five minutes away? Toilet paper is another matter.

I now insist that we have a candle or incense in the bathrooms. I just don't want our toilet area to smell like an outhouse. My wife got me a couple of nice incense burners and a couple of votive candleholders. I'm particularly fond of mountain berry candles, as well as oils and spice incense.

She says, "Easy Dick, after all it is the toilet area."

I say, "Yes, but it doesn't have to smell like a toilet area."

She says, "If it puts a smile on your face, it tickles the hell out of me."

Bless her heart, she puts up with a lot of strange stuff from me. I tell her, "Ain't love great!"

Another one of the stories my wife enjoys telling is what she calls an eating frenzy. She says a school of sharks has nothing on me, when I get into a Heath-Bar-eating-frenzy. She says the best thing to do is stay out of the way when the wrappers start flying. She was telling a friend that she was watching me unwrap heath bars and bite into them. She noticed that I was having a little trouble getting into this particular bar, so she told the friend "I was concerned. I thought he might miss a bite and take a finger off."

What can I say? I like Heath Bars.

My poker buddies wonder about some of my little quirks on occasion. We bring our own drinks to the game. The rest of the players either drink beer or water. I bring a small cooler with ice and coke and precut slices of lime. I enjoy a real Cuba libra when I play. They think it is strange to go through all the hassle of rum, coke and a squeeze of lime. I think a man should drink whatever puts a smile on his face. I will generally drink most anything. I guess it might look a little strange to see me go through the ritual of making this concoction but that's what I want, and it works for me.

If Denny had not come out of the closet, I might never have known that she is a "secret soup tureen coveter." Seeing that my wife gets every catalog known to man, and she works twelve hours a day, the two seem to conflict, but she has made time to look at all of them, by reading them as we run errands or on our way to a restaurant, or just any time we get into the car. I tend to be the driver. She says, "Look at this—is that the neatest soup tureen you have ever seen?"

I said, "What? I've never seen an interesting soup tureen. Do you mean to tell me we have been married for this long and I didn't know you had a thing for big chili bowls?"

She said, "I'll disregard that remark coming from the guy who has 'The Dragon Collection' that ate Spring, Texas. I have two soup tureens now. I won't justify another."

I said, "Wait till we hit the lottery; we'll have a whole wing in our house just for soup tureens."

I can't read a book without underlining words I don't know or have forgotten the meaning. I then put the page number in the front of the book; when I'm finished with the book, it goes on my desk to translate into my vocabulary file. I also keep a dictionary where I highlight these words. When I find a word that is already marked in this dictionary I mentally hang myself by my thumbs for five minutes, repeating the word over and over. If I find that I have highlighted and marked the word before, well, what I do is just not suitable to tell in this piece. Keep in mind the object is to remember the word and its meaning, not to punish myself.

I have also had a lot of fun by saving quotes. I underline them and save it in my quote file. Dr. Claudia Osborn got me started doing this with her book *Over My Head*. Her comment on Easter egg hunts was more than I could stand. As I mentioned before, she had a serious bike-auto accident. She came out of it with a cognitive impairment and does a fantastic job of telling folks what it was like coping with these problems as a doctor. If you haven't read her book, you need to.

When I look at my collection of quotes, it tickles me. To me it is like saving the *créme de la créme* from the books I have read. I wish I had started this with the first book I ever read. That is something else I have learned. Don't beat yourself up for something you did or did not do yesterday or yesteryear. Remember it and learn by it. I have taken the pleasure of sprinkling some of my favorite quotes liberally throughout this book.

NAPS

I give naps their own heading because I have not been able to get away from naps. This line says it better than anything else:

"I'm tired of being tired."

It makes no difference what the event might be—pool, poker, darts, eating, or even making love. If I'm tired, I have to lie down. As you can imagine, this gets old fast. It is almost like having a bell go off in my head. Ding, you're tired; go take a nap. It doesn't seem to make any difference whether I had ten hours sleep or four hours sleep the night before. If I don't get a nap, I get unbelievably grouchy. That flooding feeling gets more intense. I flood with less information coming into my mind. If the information is negative, the flooding is worse. I get things mixed up, it is difficult to concentrate. My flexibility factor is zero. I won't even try to do multi-tasking. My frustration fuse is shorter than usual. Then I get angry. At that point, I'm not fit for human company. Then with the frustration and anger feeding on each other, I find it difficult to close my eyes so that I can take a nap. My communications are poor. In short, if I don't take a nap at this point, believe me, no one wants to be around me. I'm better off going to a place to be alone to work this out. Until I come up with some kind of substitute for naps, I'll be a *napper*. I wish I could come up with something I could do while napping, maybe learning through osmosis? I believe I tried that in high school; I tried sleeping with my history book under my pillow. I still failed American history and world history and had to make them up in summer school. I'll keep working on this nap challenge.

LIDS, CAPS, STOPPERS AND TOPS

B.S. Before Surgery, I was collecting tops of things. Now I am obsessive about it. I don't mean I would pick an interesting top from the street, but I have picked them out of our trash. One day I am going to get into art, and I have decided that I will do collages with container tops. The rule is there can be no writing on the top. I have a thirty-nine gallon trash bag that is full of lids and tops. I have even saved the L'eggs containers from when Denny wore those stockings. I also have several hundred little blue caps from filters when my wife was quitting smoking. My feeling is that these will make great eyes for fish when I start doing artsy-crafty stuff. Even though I started this BS, I have a greater lid/top awareness now, AS (after surgery). Who knows, someday I may have a piece hanging in a gallery near you. At any rate, this is on my 'I want, I wish' list. This is the intermittent stop to get on the goals list. A thirty-nine gallon trash bag holds a lot of lids and caps. I could put a collage in every major art museum in the world. I think big, anyway. I've got to do the first one *first*. But then again, who would have thought that I would have two books written now? So I have faith in myself. I'll get a collage or two done, just as I have written two books.

I'm pleased to report that I am not the only one in this house who has a fetish. Denny insists that the kitchen sink be immaculate at all times. Therefore I take it as my personal challenge to see that the sink is *4.0* at all times (military talk for perfect). If I walk by and see that there is a water stain, I will pull a paper towel and wipe it out. I'm not the only one with a bathroom fetish. My wife insists that the toilet area be spotless. If I were to stand just a bit too far away and with a short horn and all, I might dribble a drop on the floor or the porcelain. Or maybe a hair might fall in the area. I wouldn't dream of leaving the bathroom without cleaning it up. You would be surprised how much of a shine you can get on porcelain if you put a little work into it. As best I can, I am a Denny supporter in as many things as I can handle. If I can do something that puts a smile on her face, it tickles me to no end. I know she feels the same way about me. Ain't love grand?

Here is a lesson for you, gentlemen. When I approach the toilet to go, I think to myself, "All right, I'll position myself so that if I dribble, I will dribble into the center of the bowl. Any hair or dribbles will be *flushable*, then I won't have to clean up afterwards."

Now pay close attention, guys. Next I'm going to teach you how to break wind politely. There will be a test of sorts.

CHOCOLATE FREAK

I could have put this under the poker section, but I think it fits better here. My wife is on a lifelong quest to find the best chocolate cookie in the world. This wasn't brought to my attention until I started playing poker at Steve's Rock & Poker Parlor. Talking to my wife the next day after my first event there, I mentioned to her that Teddy, the guy who invited me to the game, brought cookies. I thought it was kind of strange, but then again I enjoy a cookie with my whisky once in a while. These guys are mostly construction guys of one flavor or another, big burly men.

The next time Denny and I went grocery shopping, we spent a lot of time on the cookie aisle. She purchased several boxes of chocolate chip cookies. Then she told me about her never ending quest. She said she didn't buy many before because if she didn't like them she didn't want them to go to waste. Now, if they are not her favorites, she gives them to me to take to the game. It is strange to walk into the game and the players say, "Hey Dick, what's the cookie of the day?"

I say, "Chocolate chip."
Mike says, "Oh goodie, that's one of my favorites."
Strange but true.

BEARD POWER

This could actually be put in with fetish, except I feel so strongly about it I'm giving it a little section of its own. I have worn a beard most of my adult life. A.S. (After Surgery) I'm not sure how many interviews - thirty, forty - I got to thinking maybe beards are out. In my not-so-clear thinking, I shaved it clean off. I didn't care for the look even though people who have known me for a long time said it knocked fifteen years off my appearance. I couldn't stand it. I felt naked, undressed, not whole, not me. A gal told me, "Don't grow your beard back. Beards have a negative connotation—you know—Blackbeard, Bluebeard, Rasputin, Ivan The Terrible. Besides, you're a handsome man; don't hide it."

I grew my beard back. I would say to this person now, "What about Jesus, Santa, Uncle Sam, Abe? These guys have a fairly respectable reputation and image."

I will never be naked in the face again. I don't know who that other guy without the beard was, but it wasn't me.

HEROES

I have two unusual heroes I try to model myself after, as far as their personalities are concerned.

Wile E. Coyote, in the Roadrunner cartoons. I think Wile E. is the epitome of persistence. He tries everything to catch the roadrunner, misses, and goes back and tries something else. As long as he doesn't quit, he doesn't lose. I think like he does. If it is important to me "I will never, never give up."

My other unlikely hero is J. Thaddeus Toad, of Toad Hall, in The *Wind In The Willows*. My affirmation on this is "I have the courage to try new and adventurous things." To quote Thaddeus in his adventures he says, "Come, I'll show you the world." My thoughts exactly, for an adventure. Thaddeus and his pal, a horse named Cyril, went from adventures in a horse drawn gypsy trailer to adventures in a motor car, to adventures in an airplane. If I were to write the next story, they would be in a rocketship, headed for outer space. "Get out of the way Star Trek." We all need ideals, heroes, and something to shoot for. This is what keeps us alive and interested in getting up the next day to meet the challenges.

Cognitively-challenged folks, particularly, need challenges and interests. If you don't have one, get one!

Airport Flooding

Think of yourself as someone who has claustrophobia. Now imagine that you have been thrown into a coffin with a dead person in there. Then the coffin is dropped into a cave that no one knows about. That is the feeling I had when I lost my wife at the airport. She was taking me on a trip to Mexico. I was driving at this point so I let her off at the entrance to the ticketing area, so she could get the necessary paperwork taken care of and I was to meet her at the departure gate. Then we would sit and have an iced tea while we waited for boarding.

I parked the car and went into the terminal. I checked the flight and found the proper gate number and headed that way. When I got to the gate, she was nowhere to be found. I could feel the adrenaline start to rise in my system. I thought well, she hasn't finished with the paperwork yet. I started running back to the ticketing area. When I got there: no Denny. I really started to panic. You must realize that there was nothing I could do to control the feeling at that time. I knew she wouldn't leave without me, but it didn't matter.

I knew this airport well. I've flown out of there hundreds of times. The feeling persisted; I was anxious, concerned, worried, but mostly scared to death. I couldn't tell you what I was afraid of, I was just afraid. I checked the gate number again to make sure I had it right. I did. Could I have missed her while I was rechecking the flight and gate number? Maybe so. I ran back to the gate, then back to the ticketing area. Nothing! I stopped an airline employee and asked how I could page someone. I must have looked a wreck. The agent said "Oh yes, right over there. Are you all right?"

I wasn't all right, but I wasn't going to stop and tell this person. I was off and running again. I had them page my wife to meet me at this spot. I waited for a bit but to no avail. I ran to the gate again. The feeling of helplessness was overwhelming. What could I do next? I'd done everything I could think of. A line from a Dean Koontz book covered my feelings quite well at this point. "I was like a boiler with a jammed release valve, filled to the bursting point not with steam pressure but with manic terror." Then as I was walking back to the paging area I saw her coming out of the ladies room. I ran up to her, grabbed her and said, "Don't ever do that again."

She said, "What? Go to the bathroom?"

It was too soon after my surgery for me to see the humor in this. I was still puffing, panting and panicky. We had a very long talk on what I had just been through, and we agreed that we would set meeting places in case we ever got separated again. To this day, anytime we go somewhere there is the least chance we could get away from each other, we look around for a place we could meet. If I never have that stark fear again, it would be great. There is no such thing as getting used to this degree of horror, so we work very hard to keep my adrenaline flow to a minimum. I'm sure the adrenaline shoots to the top of my head; that must be why I have a bald spot like a monk's skullcap.

WORKING WITH MY HANDS

This event happened BS (Before Surgery). It is important to note that some things don't change. A good number of years ago I ran a poker game out of my house. The rule was no drinks or food on the table. The TV trays I had seen around were too small as far as I was concerned. You couldn't put an ashtray, drink, pack of cigarettes, lighter, sandwich and a bowl of nuts on one of these standard trays and use it without great difficulty.

I don't like ashes in my nut bowl any more than I like ashes or beer on my sandwich. This put me on a quest to find large TV trays. I had gone to all the standard type of stores to fulfill this mission, with no luck. One day I found myself in Neiman-Marcus at the Galleria on another matter. On my way out I was going through their kitchen supply area and, wouldn't you know it, there they were, exactly what I was looking for. The problem was they were fifty bucks apiece. I wasn't going to pay fifty dollars to have poker players burn holes in them or have some drunk sit on one. So I picked up a tray, noted the construction, made some notes and said to myself, "I can make these things for a lot less than that."

I was excited—a long time quest was about to be resolved. I stopped at a hardware store on the way home and bought the wood and hardware necessary to build four large TV trays. A week or so later, I looked to see what I had accomplished. I had built four trays at a cost of about sixty dollars apiece. Three of them were so rickety and wobbly I had to throw them away. The remaining tray would function all right, but it looked so tacky that I wouldn't have it in the house. I was embarrassed about the poor workmanship. My thoughts were that I should either have purchased the good trays or told the players to bring their own. This project confirmed something my wife knew and I suspected: this type of work was not for me.

AS (After Surgery) when I get the urge to do this type of thing, whether it be for therapy or for real, I need to remember that fiasco, and make a reindeer or two (I make yarn reindeer to give away at Christmas). It doesn't cost nearly as much and the frustration factor is much lower. So you see, we brain-damaged folks can learn. It's just that sometimes we have to pay for it. I have all the tools and I know how to use them. Somehow I just can't get that from my brain to my hands.

If God were to speak to me and say, "Dick, I want you to build an ark," we'd be in deep doo-doo.

ANGER

I was mad at myself and mad at God, even though I had no choice about getting a tumor (and I really don't think it was God's plan, either).

Why the devil can't I remember things?

What happened to my vocabulary?

Why is it every time I'm doing a task I keep forgetting what I'm doing?

Why am I always so tired?

Why can't I remember jokes anymore? I used to have a repertoire of some fifty or so jokes.

I want to be a breadwinner. I want to hit all the islands in the Caribbean and have a piña-colada tasting contest with myself. I want my wife never to have to worry about money again.

Enough crying and moping. Now I do a little positive self-talk. Anger is an enemy; don't let it be in control. I lose if anger gets the upper hand. I will be in control because I am a winner—I have a positive attitude that guarantees success.

That's okay, Dick. Wishing and wanting is the first step in figuring out how to get what you wish and want. I'm still trying to learn that when you're given lemons, you make lemonade.

When I took this not-so-advanced thought and applied it to my situation, this is what I came out with: "If you're given brain damage, write about it." Hopefully this book will give somebody an idea of how to help themselves or someone they love. And that gains momentum and the world is a better place.

ANGER: A HISTORY

I put in this little piece to show what kind of person I was as a kid and how I grew. As an adult, I have been able to maintain my cool—reasonably well. As a kid, I didn't do so well. There was a time when I was upset with a boy who was older and bigger. He was teasing me and I couldn't stand it anymore. I knew he was too tough to beat straight up so my plan was to pull the water fountain out of the ground in the park and hit him with it. (Reading this makes me think this tumor started a long time ago.)

Anger falls in with all those other negative emotions like depression and indecision; they all feed off each other. Frustration and anger have learned to play well together because they run around together. It is like having a cold and sneezing and getting a sore nose because of it. When I get frustrated, I get angry. Maybe because I can't do that "thing" anymore, that "thing" I used to do so well. Or I can't remember a word, a name or a procedure. I can't tell you how many times I would have trashed my computer. Or while talking to my health insurance people I wanted to reach through the phone and tear out their lungs, or maybe grab these non-cooperative dolts by their tongues and snap them inside out. After they were inside out, I would sit them down and say, "There, now, don't you wish you would have helped a person in need... me?" In the end I settle for "Be thankful, Dick. There are some who don't have a computer or an insurance company to complain about."

Many times I have gone back to that old proverb: "I felt bad for myself because I had no shoes, till I met the man who had no feet." If you could come with me to rehab, you would see just what I mean. Every time I look at my problems, then look at what some of my fellow rehabbers put up with, I shame myself for being so self-centered.

I'm Really Smokin' Now

I don't use tobacco or nicotine in any form. I don't smoke it, chew it, snort it or rub it on my belly. I do however smoke *Spiceys* (my term). You think that is a strange first line for a chapter with this title? Read on and see if any of this rings a bell for you or a loved one. For you folks who are hooked on nicotine, this may be a health salvation without all the folderol. No patches, gum, or withdrawal. If nothing else, I hope I give you a chuckle or two.

I started smoking seriously when I was seventeen, a senior in high school. By seriously, I mean going as far as to buy my own cigarettes (when I had the money, or borrow one out of Mom's purse if she wasn't around).

In those days you could buy a pack of Luckies out of a machine for twenty-five cents. With that you got three shiny pennies under the cellophane and a book of matches. (It was like a starter kit.) I've seen people buy out of the machines these days and their arms get tired putting quarters in. Of course they are so expensive the manufacturer was kind enough to put slots for dollar bills. And of course the cigarette manufacturers wouldn't dream of spending the extra money to include matches in this exorbitant price. Why should they? They know you're hooked and you will find your own light. And you will find it fast, if they know their smoking market, and they do.

Speaking of hooked, for more years than I care to mention the last thing I did every night was to have a cigarette. I would put it out and roll over and go to sleep. The first thing I did every morning was light one up. I mean the very first thing. Also I might add, it was not unusual for me to get up two or three times in the middle of the night and have a smoke or two. How's that for being addicted?

This wouldn't be a story about smoking if I didn't talk about burning holes in clothes. I happen to be a convertible person. I've been driving a convertible of one sort or another for a good number of years and every one of them had cigarette burns somewhere. Of course, the classic is dropping your cigarette or a hot ash in your lap while you're driving in traffic. That's good for at least a hole in your pants, if not a hole in the car seat. As you are driving around digging at your crotch, diligently trying to recapture this wild ash, the people around you are saying, "Look at that pervert," or thinking "I'll bet he dropped a live cigarette."

I'm not sure how many shirts, pants, sport coats, and suits I threw away because I had burned holes in them by dropping the hot ashes in my lap, or having the cigarette in my mouth and lifting my arm for whatever reason, then turn my head. Zap, there goes another hole. If it were a favorite shirt or jacket, I would consider having a re-weave done, but, as you may know, these are very expensive. If I had all the money back I've spent on repairing cigarette burn holes, I'm sure I could buy a round of drinks for Spring, Texas.

I tried smoking corn silk as a young kid. At that point I sure couldn't tell why adults enjoyed smoking. Although it was very alluring to watch my uncles blow smoke rings; it looked like fun to me. Smoking corn silk was a little like my first taste of bourbon. I didn't know why on earth anybody would want to put their throat through that kind of torture. It just made no sense to me. Smoking corn silk was like swallowing a porcupine against the grain. I tried smoking cigarettes several times and each time I got sicker than the time before. I think God was trying to tell me something. You would think that anybody who threw up as violently as I did during these experiments would say, "Okay, that's not for me." You would also think that being down on all fours retching and seeing what I believed to be my stomach lying there in the grass would be enough for any sane person, even a young person, to say *enough already.*

Then a couple of days might pass and I would see someone looking like they were really enjoying an after dinner smoke. Or I would go to a movie and see the really cool guys smoking. I'm thinking, *if I want to be cool I've got to smoke.*

Well anyway, some of the guys I hung around with started smoking in the sixth grade. It just took me a little longer to get the hang of it.

One of the things I always found fascinating is where a person kept his cigarettes. For a while in high school it was cool to roll them in the sleeve of your T-shirt. This served several purposes. This showed the teachers that you were a rebel to be reckoned with, as well as showing the girls you were cool, just like Marlon Brando in *The Wild One* or James Dean in *Rebel Without A Cause*. That whole scene got old after a while and I just put them in a pocket. In the shirt was okay; in the Levis you ended up with flat cigarettes. But they still smoked.

After high school and before the Navy, a friend of mine and I went to the wilds of British Columbia, Canada to pan gold. This was a unique experience for several reasons. I ran out of smokes and my friend and I traveled fifty miles to get to a small place called Hope, BC. As small as the town was, they did have a general store that handled cigarettes. Not being familiar with Canadian cigarettes, I just asked the clerk for some smokes. She gave me a cigarette by the name of Black Cats. This is where I first became aware of the term **bridge tobacco**. For you people who are unaware of this term, I will explain. There is this covered bridge, like in the movie *Legend of Sleepy Hollow,* that is a main thoroughfare for horse and carriage traffic. Of course, as the horses go through they kick up splinters of wood, urinate and drop horse apples. The next horse that goes through the bridge mixes up what the previous horses have left behind and so on. This leaves a mixture of wood splinters, horse urine, and horse poop. Now once a month or so this guy comes along with a broom and dust pan, sweeps this stuff up and sells it to some cigarette manufacturer. This is called bridge tobacco. Now I'm not saying that the people who manufacture Black Cat cigarettes are users of bridge tobacco. However, when I smoked these things, I would say to my friend, "All right now, I'll hold the gun on you and you can get your nicotine fix."

Harsh tasting didn't near cover the term for the taste of these things. I think Black Cat cigarettes are the reason people talk about how tough Canadian lumberjacks are. I've heard tell these guys don't shave, they just hit themselves in the face with the flat of the ax, drive the whiskers in, then chew them off from the inside and spit them out. This would be a piece of cake after smoking a Black Cat or two.

Several years in the Navy showed me some new tricks. The Navy is also where I found out the value of Zippo lighters. They would light under most circumstances. You also had the joy of over-filling the lighter with fluid, then having it leak in your pocket. This promoted a severe rash on your leg and of course made you smell like a napalm bomb. Now by regulation, if you were in dress uniform you put the cigarettes in your sock. That worked reasonably well, except in the summer I would sweat, and end up with soggy cigarettes. When the Chief Petty Officer said, "If you've got 'em, smoke 'em," they were soggy, but they still smoked.

I spent a good deal of my youth working around the world. Part of this time I spent as a steel worker, specifically as a bridge painter. This posed some unique problems for the smoker. Because we were painting with a lead based paint, we had to wear several layers of clothes to avoid lead poisoning. We also wore heavy work gloves for the same reason. Now when you're a couple of hundred feet above the ground, covered from head to toe in green paint and starting to go into nicotine withdrawal, you start pawing around trying to remember where you put the cigarettes. My first attempt at trying to keep cigarettes paint-free and round was to use a plastic case that would hold my cigarettes as well as a book of matches. Then I would stick this package in any pocket. I still found that the smokes would get some paint on them, just in the process of getting them out and lighting them, and it was a slow, tedious job to get to them. After all, I wanted a nicotine fix NOW. I finally ended up just putting them in my pocket. With all the green bridge paint I smoked, not to mention the red lead, I am amazed that I never got lead poisoning.

There was a British cigarette called "English Ovals." After sitting on a pack of cigarettes for a few hours, they became flat (ovalish). We bridge-painters called these "Green Ovals." If you believe there is something exciting about smoking a flat green cigarette two-hundred feet in the air that tasted like paint, you too are in need of psychiatric help.

As long as I am covering smoking I guess I should throw in a story about smoking pot. That is marijuana or cannabis or any of the other zillion street names. My bumming around took me to New York City. At this point I was traveling with a very hip chick, and we were visiting her sister and her sister's boyfriend who had a loft near Battery Park. I was twenty-one years old and had never tried marijuana. I had been afraid to try it because I was under the impression that if you took one puff you would be a dope addict for the rest of your life, however short that may be. I watched the three of them pass a joint around and get goofy. They convinced me that I would not turn into a junkie for just trying it. The boyfriend said he would teach me all about pot and pot smoking. I was an eager learner. I tried smoking a joint, using a bong, several kinds of water pipes with several different kinds of liquids in them. I didn't feel a thing.

I said to him, "How long does it take to get high on this stuff? I could get higher holding my breath."

We went out for a walk in Battery Park. I looked off in the distance and saw this large building, I said, "What is that?"

He said, "That's the United Nations building."

It looked like one big window all lit up to me. Shortly after that I found myself on all fours puking my guts out and looking at my stomach lying there in the grass again. Later I found that you can't see the UN building from Battery Park. Looking back, I wonder what *he* was smoking. You would think that with the trouble I have had putting foreign substances into my body I had learned not to do that any more. Not so!

After traveling around the world and having smoked cigarettes from all over, I finally settled in Washington, D.C. The city of Washington, D.C. is a very heavy partying town. I mention this just for you folks who have never tipped your beer back to get a good long slug, only to find at the end of your chug-a-lug you have a cigarette butt in your mouth. Believe me this is enough to make you give up drinking and smoking (almost).

I was sharing an apartment with a guy named Bruce, who also enjoyed smoking a little grass now and again. We decided that the price to buy the stuff was exorbitant, so we would grow our own. We had a second floor apartment with plenty of sun, so we planted some seeds in a planter and ended up with one marijuana plant. We nurtured it, watered it, and fed it African violet food. The plant prospered and grew to be about four foot high; it never got any taller because we couldn't resist sampling the goods. We would pick leaves off, dry them out in the oven and then smoke them. For some reason this stuff tasted mentholated. We decided it was the African violet food that caused this flavor but we could never duplicate the taste with our other horticultural experiments. We couldn't resist giving our grass-smoking friends a taste. The plant never did reach maturity but it was the topic of many a conversation. We felt if we could market mentholated pot, it would be our first million dollar endeavor.

About this same time Bruce heard from some reliable source (probably a chick who had not drawn a sober breath in years) that smoking bananas peels was another non-addictive high. It's too bad we didn't have the sense to buy stock in Chiquita; we certainly must have driven it up considerably. We tried smoking the peels, raw first. Trying to set fire to a raw banana skin is almost impossible. Note I say *almost*, but we could not get the desired effect. We put the peels in a blender, chopped 'em, pureed 'em, baked 'em, fried 'em, dried them with a heat lamp, and dried them in the sun. Then we smoked this stuff. Still nothing. As I said before, we could get higher holding our breath. Part of our problem was getting rid of the by-product, in this case, the meat of the banana. You can have bananas only so many ways. To this day, when I hold a banana in my hand my gag reflex kicks in just a bit and my stomach jumps and says, *oh no, not again*. My conscience tells me, "What? You want to see your stomach lying there on the ground again?" I think the Chiquita banana people started the rumor about a new natural high.

At this point in my life I became a salesperson and later a lobbyist. Both of these professions call for alot of phone work. I would find that I might have two or three cigarettes going at the same time. Or maybe light them, put them in an ashtray and let them burn up. If I didn't know better I would say that the cigarette makers invented the telephone. Even though I let the cigarettes burn down in an ashtray, I still needed my nicotine fix, so I would light another one.

After several years of partying and drinking my share of beers with butts in them, I found the woman I love. It so happened she also smoked. Ah, but a different brand. We decided we would smoke one kind of cigarette, so we bought several kinds of filter cigarettes, then we had a blind taste test in the bathroom with the lights out to see what would be our brand. As it ended up we really didn't care, as long as we got the nicotine fix. So we ended up smoking Raleighs for the coupons. Our reasoning was sound. "As long as we smoke, let's get some added value out of this." We moved to Texas and for several years we smoked this brand. We got stuff like toasters or irons with the coupons, and we were lucky if the devices we got from the coupons lasted through the next carton of cigarettes.

One day my wife had a revelation: she said, "All this smoking is not good for our health. I'm giving it up." She had one more cigarette and said, "That's my last one." This was the ultimate in cold turkey. She is tough. That was many years ago, and she hasn't had so much as a puff since.

Ten or so years later, I looked back to discover that for the most part of the last thirty-five years I had smoked two to four packs a day, depending on what I was doing. Playing poker or out drinking with the boys was always the worst; it would be a lead-pipe cinch that day was going to be a four packer.

I'm not a health nut, although I guess I should be. Somewhere around the time frame I had emergency brain surgery is also the period that I established a new life-long credo: *Always be concerned about quality of life*. The brain surgery thing showed me that you could be taken off this earth at any time, for any reason. I decided I would give up putting nicotine into my body, but I would not give up smoking. As far as I was concerned smoking was a part of my *Quality of life*. I wasn't anxious to give up blowing smoke rings, or all the to-dos I go through to get a cigarette lit and in my mouth and ready to smoke. It was almost like a religious ceremony.

I decided that we would paint the inside of the house and turn it into a non-smoking home. After all, everyone else in our supper club and bridge group have no smoking houses. I almost upchucked when I started doing the pre-cleaning for painting.

The pictures above my chair were outlined on the wall with a brown mook that was sticky and smelled. If you want to give yourself a reason to give up smoking, take a couple of pictures off your wall and see what you have left. Ugh!

I decided I would ease myself away from the demon tobacco with its various poisons, additives and addictive substances. Who knows what they are putting into cigarettes these days? The cigarette manufacturers freely admit to adding more nicotine and some *other* stuff.

My first thought is, "I'll go to a tobacconist and see what he recommends." Don't look at this as going to a drug pusher and asking, "What do you carry that won't kill me or get me hooked?" Look at it more as though I'm going to a candy shop and saying to the proprietor, "What else do you have? I'm allergic to the last candy I got here and it made me sick." I found out there are many brands of tobacco cigarettes that are all natural products. Don't get me wrong: they still have tobacco and nicotine, just not all the other junk manufacturers put in them to preserve the flavor and get you hooked on the cancer sticks. As it turned out I ended up going to a head shop for advice. For the uninformed, this is a shop that caters to dope paraphernalia papers, pipes, screens, etc. They had a much better selection of natural tobacco cigarettes as well as cigarettes with no tobacco or nicotine.

I went about changing my smoking habit much like I used to do a sales campaign on a new market. I realized that sucking any foreign material into my lungs was not good for me. I wanted to reduce the intake as much as possible, but still try to keep some flavor. I purchased a cigarette holder that had a filter in it. I also bought a cigarette case. I decided on a cigarette that was a blend of ginseng and all natural tobacco. I bought what I considered to be my last carton of coffin nails and a carton of the new ginseng things. I would fill my cigarette case with half ginseng and half poison things. Every time I filled my case I would change filters in my cigarette holder. I figured this would be a good way to slip into my new smoking role. And it was! After finishing those two cartons, my next step was to integrate myself into no nicotine at all. There are numerous cigarettes that have no nicotine at all. The head shops and tobacconists have catalogs full of these types, as well as bulk herbs and spices for those of you who want to roll your own. A rolling machine is optional.

I had kicked the habit of all the artificial junk they put in, and it was no great shakes at all. Now to ease myself away from nicotine, the foulest poison of them all, I mixed one last carton of all natural tobacco cigarettes with my new herbs and spices. After one go 'round with this, I was ready to give up nicotine altogether. It was definitely a feeling of freedom. I could now give up smoking altogether or just go with the herbs and spices, which I call *Spiceys*. For my quality of life I still wanted to blow smoke rings. So I kept on with the *Spiceys*.

I decided on a brand called Kickum. Rather apropos, wouldn't you say? They come in three flavors: spice, menthol or originals. The blend in these cigarettes is a mixture of different herbs and spices. The primary spices are jasmine, chamomile, broom flowers, clove, damiana, sage, coltsfoot, wild lettuce, peppermint, and thyme. Almost sounds healthy, doesn't it? Now when I filled my cigarette case, it was with Kickums and the all natural tobacco cigarettes. No additives at all, thank you.

To give you an idea of other choices for *Spiceys,* here are some other spices that are mixed in with different non-nicotine smokes: catnip, passion flower, mint, love and light, ginseng, corn silk, yerba santa, licorice, mullein, horehound, marshmallow, red clover, althaea, and khatmi. So you see, if you're really serious about getting the nicotine monkey off your back, you have lots of choices.

You still need to be careful. Ann, my dart playing friend is terribly allergic to cloves. I couldn't smoke clove *Spiceys* in her presence. She would go into a sneezing attack.

Be a considerate person.

I was on vacation in Aruba, sitting at the bar. I lit a *Spicey*, and got a look from the bartender that said we don't want your kind in here. One of the people at the bar said I'll trade you one of my cigarettes for one of yours. They *do* smell somewhat like grass. The manager of the hotel came over and actually made me prove that I was smoking herbs and spices and not marijuana. I discovered that the *Spiceys* are a great conversation starter.

For your quality of life you may choose to get totally clean. Take nothing into your lungs but air. Of course you know if you live in a big city there's no telling what other substances you are inhaling as well. Most important, you are not hooked on nicotine anymore. I'm now smoking less than a pack a day of the *Spiceys*, and enjoying smoking more than ever and even though these *Spiceys* are quite expensive, about twenty dollars a carton, they should be exempt from the up and coming tobacco tax. (Don't get excited, the government will come up with some kind of tax.)

I am still blowing smoke rings, getting all the oral gratification I need, and I still have my smoking ritual. But I am nicotine-free. In short, I am smoking less and enjoying it more.

A Tool To Use, A Strategy

I am blessed with having taste buds that go wild now and again.

Denny says, "Dick, I know your taste buds were shot off in the war and they replaced them with plastic ones."

That may be, but there are certain things that every now and then taste remarkably yummy and I may eat a lot of them and do it frequently. Some of my all-time favorites have been Nibs licorice, chocolate Necco wafers, and Heath bars.

Do you remember when Nibs came in a box that had a window? On the box itself were pyramids and camels. For my money they had the true taste of licorice. Nibs was my benchmark for licorice.

I'll bet you my best huntin-hound against your hat that the recipe has been changed. I still eat Nibs, but I say they're not as good as they used to be and now that the old ones are gone, the taste has become legendary to me.

Or, you can go along with what my wife tells me, that my taste buds were shot off in the war.

Or, that I lost a little of my gourmet appreciation when they took a nip out of my gray-matter.

In high school Fran Selje, the man who introduced me to belly laughs, (now deceased; I miss you already) used to slide the Neccos down a bannister of one flight of stairs. I would be on the next flight down and catch them in my mouth, like a giant dragon snapping skiers out of the sky as they were coming off the world's biggest sky jump. Fun at the time. I wonder what kind of bugs and diseases I caught off that railing. Someone told me once that we all eat a bushel basket full dirt before we die. The powers-that-be must have allotted me a tad more.

I was also into Jelly Bellies and gum drops for awhile. There were more, but they slip my mind right now. My latest thing is popsicles. I like them all, all flavors and brands, but my present favorite is the blue raspberry from Kroger.

It was Friday and we always shopped on Saturday, so I had Friday night to contend with, as far as noshes were concerned. Denny was busy with e-mail and voice mail. This has been known to take three or four hours so I have in mind that I will buy a box of popsicles to hold me over till the next day. When I got to the store freezer, I saw a sign that said "3 boxes for $5.00". I know they will never go to waste, so I bought three boxes. On the way home, I got to thinking, what does this habit cost us? My mind starts to leap into math. Let's see, five bucks for three boxes. There is a confusion factor here, on the box it says "Not twelve, but sixteen." But it is still the same old five bucks. Don't forget the Governor. He gets thirty-eight cents or so. That's five thirty-eight. Was that twelve or sixteen? Oh yes, sixteen popsicles per box. Now do I want to divide sixteen into five thirty-eight, then divide by three? Or do I want to multiply three times sixteen then divide that into five thirty-eight. What the devil is three times sixteen anyway? Now my mind took a big leap and went to darts, not my choice, it just went there. Three sixteens happens a lot. Three sixteens is forty-eight points. It struck me as strange, I didn't think of this as math, I thought of it as darts. But the problem got solved. Now I slipped back into math. Forty-eight into five thirty-eight is…this isn't rocket science. Fifty into five bucks is, ten cents a popsicle. Even a brain-damaged dude can work that out. The point being that some synapses got crossed. I got some cost per box, mixed it with my darts and it worked beautifully. Maybe bowlers, ball players, marble shooters or water skiers, or maybe even yo-yo players can find something in their hobby, or their sports world or any area of their lives that they crossover to help another area. We need to free-associate more. That thought is to borrow knowledge from one area and apply it to others, and we need to get to the point that we do this automatically. I'm doing this with darts now to help me with my math. It still does not come automatically. But it's like any other tool, the more I use it the better I get with it. If I don't use it, I lose it. You too! If you haven't figured your crossover skills yet, hang in there; if you look for them they will show up.

When it happens, write it down immediately. Then tell a friend and your soul-mate or a relative exactly what happened so you won't have too much trouble recreating the event. Now that you have done it again, it is your tool to use any time you want. And yours to show to fellow rehabbers, so you can help them find their tools. Man, does that feel good.

A Broken Recognizer

My wife is a professional woman, and thank God she dresses the part. She will say, "What do you think of this new outfit?" She has come to realize that I don't tend to notice new things. She thinks it is a pattern recognition problem and she is probably right. At supper club we were all talking about giving compliments on the things our wives wore. One of the wives said, "Before Ed would tell me I looked good in a new outfit, the devil would be serving iced tea and lemonade at his lunches."

I said, "Maybe I'm not brain-damaged, I'm just a husband."

Denny gave me one of those askance looks that says, A-huh, and if you believe that, we better get you in for some additional therapy.

Trying new things, whether it might be a new restaurant, getting a new shirt, trying a previously untried short-cut, anything that might be new, is tough. Change is tough. Don't change the furniture. Don't rearrange shelves or closets.

Denny says, "Your aversion to change comes from your "terrible-twos" period, with a smidgen of rebellious teens thrown in. I don't know where she would get that idea. I'm sure I was a "little darling" whether I was two or a teen.

A broken *recognizer* comes in many forms when you are brain-damaged. One of the more embarrassing problems is putting names, faces, places and events together. Most everyone has experienced "I *know* I know that guy, but from where?"

Some people might think, "If he doesn't remember me, I guess I'm not that important to him." Please don't think that for a second. My ability to recognize people, places and things has a little hitch in it: if you help me out a few times, it will help me retain that information. That, in turn, will help me retrieve your name, face, and our relationship. If we have had a chance to chat, I want to remember you. My surgeon told my wife that when many people who have this type of operation come out of the recovery room, they don't recognize their spouses. We were lucky! I've been tempted to approach Denny and say, "Didn't I pick you up in a bar in Cleveland and we spent the weekend together?" I may be brain-damaged but I'm not stupid. We kid around a lot, but this is an area I won't play in. It is too easy to misunderstand all the meanings and ramifications if it is taken wrong.

If your recognizer is broken, work on it. Hopefully you can get some new synapses snapping and that is the road to fixing a recognizer that is on the fritz.

INSTANT GRATIFICATION

I have always been a person who wants it *now*. We planted some oleanders. My idea is that the last step I take in planting is snapping my fingers. This should automatically start the plant blooming those gorgeous deep red flowers. No matter how hard I snapped my fingers, the blooms just would not come out. You can't hurry Mother Nature.

How about looking at something that I have complete control over? I collect what I consider to be interesting quotes, as well as words that I am not familiar with and words that I knew BS (Before Surgery), but have forgotten since. I underline the word, then write the page number in the front of the book. When I finish the book I take it to my desk and sit down with my dictionary and look up the word and mark the word in the dictionary. Then I write the word into my collection along with the book title and the author. When I come to a word that is already marked, I know that I have had that word before.

The frustrating part is when I see that the word has been marked several times. I see no reason why my mind won't grasp that word so I will never forget it. But of course my mind does not work that way. I came to the word "eclectic." It had been marked four times. That is totally unacceptable; I knew that I had used the word in my everyday vocabulary Before Surgery, but it just was not sticking with me. My first thought was, how the devil can I be a writer if I can't retain and recover words, build my vocabulary and use the words? There is very little instant gratification when you are brain-damaged. Oh well, I won't give up. I guess I'm going to have to personalize everything to help me retain it; I'm still working on ways to retrieve it once I have it. *Eclectic*, made up of elements from various sources. I have an eclectic collection of dragons. They come from all parts of the world, from all sorts of people, and in all shapes, sizes and materials. If that isn't eclectic, I don't know what is. This may be a slow fingernail-biting procedure, but I will improve my vocabulary and I will retain words, and retrieve them as I need them. So there!

A problem I have found with my fellow cognitively-challenged partners is that when we don't get that instant gratification, we occasionally go off like a sky rocket. Please have patience with us, even though *we* seem to have none. My wife says my fuse is shorter than my memory, and you know how short my memory is. My retention and retrieval switch seems to be locked in the forget mode. But I am working on getting new pathways going, and new synapses snapping. Gaining new pathways and new snapping synapses is a slow and arduous task. I've talked to a lot of experts at Project ReEntry about this problem and they all say the same thing: "Slow and easy Dick, don't forget to use as many strategies as possible." That is tough for a guy who is bent toward instant gratification.

There are certain things I just can't do socially that I would like to do because it would be instant gratification. A guy got on the elevator in the Rehab Building. He was a big man and he pushed his way in and was not courteous at all. He forced a little mother and child to go to the corner, even though it was only one flight. I had to make a bowel movement something fierce and I'm afraid I let a little gas pass, very odiferous. I had to bite my tongue to keep from saying to this guy just loud enough so that everyone on the elevator could hear, "Look at me, they'll think I did it."

I'm trying to learn how to get along in polite society, so I didn't want to start a precedent of unsociable activities.

CONVALESCING AT HOME

Our insurance company, in their infinite wisdom, decided twelve days in ICU and one day in the neurology ward was sufficient for recovery. They insisted that I go home, *now*! I couldn't even go to the toilet by myself. This was just the first of many a debacle that occurred involving the medical insurance side of this event.

If I weren't already cognitively-impaired by the operation, dealing with the insurance company, the hospital and the U.S. government would surely have driven me to start blabbering to myself. I wasn't dealing well with any of this; I had an inkling that the guys in the white suits carrying the funny jackets with the wrap-around sleeves were going to come and invite me to leave with them.

I was afraid they would tell me they had a great padded cell for me, complete with catered meals. I would never hold my wife's hand nor walk a Caribbean beach again, never hear a bird sing, nor ever go to a new restaurant again. Dealing with these large entities seemed like fighting with the IRS in a no-holds-barred audit. It seemed to me they had me over a barrel and were greasing me up. They had the trump cards and could hold their breath forever. I had no control and must follow their guidelines to get anything done, and of course, all their guidelines seemed to lead me into a catch twenty-two. You can't do this until you do that. You can't do that until you establish this other thing. On and on into the bureaucratic red tape. Procedures of this type lead to maximum frustration and a tidal wave of flooding. Flooding is the bane of my existence.

Flooding takes many forms. I'll list a few now and a few later as they fit in. One of the biggest *flooders* is an excess of incoming information. I may or may not have to make decisions with this incoming information. Decision-making falls under the category of executive functioning skills. This category in general is a 'biggie' for flooding.

Decision-making now is not one of my strong suits. As a matter of fact, after I started to make decisions my wife rewarded me with *at-a-boys* of one flavor or another. Going to a favorite restaurant was high on my list of rewards. Heavy emotions came into play when I finally started making decisions. What happens if I do this, or what happens if I decide to do that? How will this all effect me? I'm flooding as I write this.

How much should I include? I don't want to overwhelm you as a reader, but on the other hand, it is imperative that you understand how frightening this stage was, and is. One form of flooding comes from information and emotional overload. It has a claustrophobic as well as a suffocating feeling.

The term flooding is *apropos*. I fight to try and get a breath, to try and understand how to handle this. I'm still working on this problem and I am told by the brain peekers (shrinks, psychologists, all of that ilk) that I can expect to go through this for the rest of my life.

I'll get a handle on it. I have to, to stay sane and beat this whole thing. It is amazing to me how all the deficits seem to play on each other. Even the being tired all the time and having to take frequent naps, or thinking about napping, leads to a form of flooding.

I say to myself, if I didn't have to nap I could get a lot more accomplished. But then if I don't nap I get tired and irritable. This makes me feel like a junk yard dog—just don't mess with me. I hate feeling like that, which, again, is a flavor of flooding. How can my wife and people around me live with me when I'm like this? I'm afraid you will see many more examples of the different iterations of flooding. This affliction shows in all aspects of my life. It sure did change my social activity, mostly negatively, and all poopy I'm afraid. (At least at first.)

Judgment went out the window as well when I lost my executive functioning skills. To give you an idea of how bad my judgment was, I wanted to drive myself home from the hospital! Judgment is something you have to build and keep a repertoire of, like when you're driving a car you look to see if there is enough room to enter a freeway where the traffic is going sixty-five miles an hour (in Houston it's more like ninety-five). After a try or two I can realize what must take place for me to get out there with the rest of the "brain-damaged" people.

Talk about denial! I thought I could pick up where the old me had left off. I was sure it was just a matter of going to an interview, then accepting the job. After two more years of total frustration and anger (this includes something on the order of seventy-five job interviews), I was still in denial. I was told this tumor could have been affecting me for the last couple of years. No wonder my work performance was not up to my standards. My interviewing skills were down the tubes. I remember I used to revel in sharing success stories. I couldn't remember how to verbalize these stories; I couldn't remember how to probe to find things out and let the interviewer see that I knew how to get answers. The entire interviewing process was nerve wracking, depressing, and demoralizing, not to mention that it caused me to flood. I felt like I was swimming up Niagara Falls every time I sat across the desk from a would-be job situation. I felt embarrassed for the person interviewing me. I felt they were saying to themselves "What is this loser doing talking to me about this high performance, high paying, high visibility position? I wouldn't let him sweep up around here."

I do my best to keep control. The more I do it the better I get at it.

MULTI-TASKING

I never thought I would hear myself say this, but it must be said that multi-tasking is a thing of the past. To break this down to its simplest form, I can't walk and chew gum very well anymore. My wife was talking to me while I made the bed before she was running to a meeting with a client. As I was making the bed she was giving me some directions on tasks she would like me to do that day and I was trying to listen to her and make the bed at the same time. When she asked me to repeat the tasks and the directions, I got it totally turned around: drop the cleaning off, pick up a prescription, deposit a check and be sure to put gas in her van. Rehab was the next day and I had already told her my gas was low, one more thing to remember to do today. I couldn't get her tasks too mixed up; after all, I certainly couldn't deposit a check at the cleaners, nor could I get gas at the bank. As I listened to her, I was trying to make a hospital fold at the foot of the bed. The message was a big jumble in my mind. The bed looked like a two-year-old was trying to hide toys under the covers. I was frustrated. Both of these are simple tasks. I stopped making the bed and reached for pen and paper on my bedside table. By the way, I always have pen and paper in the ready position. This should probably be rule number one for the cognitively-challenged. I took copious notes on the things I was to do and remade the bed after she left for her appointment. If I print *slowly* and *carefully* I can read and understand my notes later. It was a challenge for my wife to speak slowly, wait for me to write, and then double check my notes to make sure I had it correctly. At first I could tell this slow communication was frustrating to her as well as to me. Now that she has the hang of it, she is an excellent communicator.

PETS

*D*on't take on the responsibility of a pet unless you're willing to do it for the life span of the pet. Since our marriage several decades ago we have had pets and loved them. We take our pet chores and obligations seriously, and through the years we have mostly had two dogs and two cats at the same time. We have found this arrangement works well for the beasties and for us. Watching puppies and kitties play is a most gratifying event.

At this point, we have two dogs. Shardak our big dog is half collie and half shepherd. He is over a hundred pounds and is a sweetheart. Our small dog, Dancer, is a miniature poodle who was abused as a pup. She is a small tornado. We adopted both dogs from the humane society.

We have two cats, a calico we call Cali and a torty we named Wisconsin (as a kitten she looked like a badger). Wisci and Cali are litter mates and both of these cats act a bit standoffish, with some exceptions. If Denny is eating a chocolate popsicle Cali will find her. If I am working at my desk, Wisci wants to smell my hand while I am writing notes or what-have-you. I tried telling Denny that was the reason I have such bad penmanship but she is not brain-damaged and didn't buy it.

All disabled people should have pets. Every statistic we have seen shows that people with pets live longer and have fuller lives. Just having them around gives another facet to life, gets different synapses snapping. The love that is returned is of a variety that is hard to come by anywhere else.

Because Shardak's personality is so sweet we wanted to get a puppy so he could help raise it. He is eleven now. We went to the pound to look for a big dog for all of us to raise. (Cali tends to mother Shardak, so we are sure she will do the same for a new pup.) We didn't find one that wanted to come home with us so we didn't get a puppy. However, as Denny was walking by the kittens she saw a snowshoe—as a matter of fact it was a *quadra polydactyl*. The term means that the cat has extra toes on all four feet. She looked to be half Angora and half Siamese with the most beautiful blue eyes you have ever seen. Her eyes would make Paul Newman's and Frank Sinatra's look mundane. My wife latched on to that kitten and carried it around while we looked at puppies. The newest member of our menagerie is called Indigo, for obvious reasons. We're still looking for a big dog; we've given some thought to getting a Tibetan mastiff. We'll see.

I heard an animal trainer say that if we would raise our kids like we raise our pets and our pets like our kids, we would have a better bunch of each. I don't know about that, but I can tell you that we spoil our animals something fierce, and we love it. It doesn't bother Denny a wink to spend several dollars for a pet toy.

To open a gallon of milk, I had to pull this little pink pull-tab to get the lid off. I set the pink plastic pull-tab on the center cabinet. Indigo was there with me, and she started playing with it. Off she went, hitting it, chasing it, and having a great time. I in turn was having a great time watching. It turns out this is the greatest cat toy since the wind-up mouse. Indigo thought so, anyway.

This little episode made me think if she were a kid she would be playing with the box the present came in, not the present, which is another way of saying, "One man's trash is another man's treasure." I will be careful about saying things like "That's a dumb idea" or "Who would ever believe that?"

Be kind. Stepping on someone else's sacred cow could lead to eating crow. With your foot in your mouth it is tough to say, "I'm sorry, I didn't realize that was so important to you."

If you are a feeling, concerned person and you engage your mind before you engage your mouth, you can stay out of most touchy situations.

GRIEF

Shardak, our big dog, has had a skin-eating disease for the last year and this has necessitated several major operations. The elbows on his front legs are open, raw flesh; they could never be healed. His front legs require cleaning, medication and fresh bandages nightly. He has in the last four months developed arthritis so badly in his hips that I made a sling for him out of a dog seat harness and a couple of straps with buckles. He is no longer able to go outside to do his business and he lies there and soils himself. I carry him out morning, noon and night. He can't stand on his back legs. The only way he can go to the toilet is if he is lying down. And of course he ends up with feces and urine all over his stomach and backside.

My heart went out to this old diplomat. This is not quality in life. He had always been a clean beast and he was extremely alert. He just couldn't do his toiletries. My wife, bless her soul, was trying different medications, homeopathic cures and acupuncture. We were trying to find a cure for the hip ailment. After thousands of dollars, several veterinary specialists, and much advice from homeopathic specialists, we could see that he wasn't gaining any ground. His quality of life was non-existent. My wife and I agree that life without quality is not worth living. Our vet, Dr. Drow, is only ten minutes from the house. I couldn't call to let them know I was bringing Shardak in to be sent to Valhalla (another name for heaven, as I understand it.) Every time I picked the phone up to call I started crying. I just could not control it. Finally my wife saw the problem and called the vet to let them know I was bringing my dog in. On the way over to the vet's I kept my hand on Shardak, petting him and telling him he was going to meet our other animals who have died, and then I named them all. I told him between gasps of crying that I loved him. That was one of the toughest things I ever had to do. The pain was immense, and I had absolutely no control.

The day after I put Shardak down, my wife and I were having lunch and I said, "I want to make a toast to the big dog." She was drinking iced tea, while I was having a beer.

She said, "I don't think Shardak would mind if I toasted him with a soft drink, do you?"

I said, "It's not the spirit in your glass that counts. It's the spirit in your heart and soul that counts. Here's to Shardak, the big dog."

Trying not to cry, I focused on the positives: we were incredibly lucky to have had a dog like Shardak, his disposition was exactly like I would have designed it. I thought of all the good times we'd had together, and I cried again and again.

Mining For Kitty-gold

Cleaning the kitty litter is now one of my responsibilities. I have to keep a cheery outlook when I do this because it is not one of my favorite jobs. Denny keeps the kitty boxes in her office, so I want to be sure they are as clean as possible and make sure I get all the little gold nuggets. I do have a bit of a challenge in her office once in a while because Dancer, our purple 'poodelope,' likes to stop by Denny's office for a snack of kitty-gold. When she snacks, she is very messy; kitty litter and what-have-you will be found all around. Every morning and every night, I vacuum her office with one of those battery operated jobs. While I have the vacuum in my hand I walk the rest of the house, searching out little pieces of stuff the dogs may have dragged in. It sure makes for a cleaner house. If there is ever a market for kitty or dog waste, I believe we can corner that market.

Every now and again Priscilla, the gal in charge of the intensive care unit when I was having brain surgery, watches our menagerie, two cats and two dogs, when we are called to the Caribbean for healing. When she is called away on business, or takes a vacation, she allows me to mine kitty-gold at her house. I might also mention that Priscilla has two entries in the "Dragon Collection that Ate Texas." Have you ever seen a bearded, beaded dragon? Neither had I until Priscilla traded me the dragon for the kitty-gold. I thought it was a heck of deal, but I'm going to keep an eye on her: *she* may corner the market for kitty-gold! I could get wealthy; we have three cats now, and I'll get another if the kitty-gold market goes up. It is amazing how proficient even a brain-damaged guy can get at searching for kitty-gold when he does it a couple of times a day. Priscilla's newest entry is a glass-blown Red Dragon of Wales and it's a beaut!

I am the best kitty-gold-miner in Spring, Texas, as I always strive to be the best I can at whatever I am engaged in, whether it is mining kitty-gold or learning a new word.

PATIENCE & FRUSTRATION

When I run out of patience, as with many things that I might run out of, the next thing I run into is frustration. Ah yes, the joys of having a nick taken out of your gray matter. There are a few things in life that call for patience. Waiting for undesirable things to stop is one of them. Like passing a dead skunk on the road: you know the smell is going to stop in a moment or two. The kid scraping his fingernails on a chalkboard or maybe somebody babbling tripe in a conversation, the aftertaste in your mouth when you take an unpleasant medicine, the pain in your finger when you burn it on a match or hot iron till you put an ice cube on it. Certainly this type of irritation can take place with all the senses.

My wife and I decided we would go to one of our favorite restaurants. Carrabba's has one of the finest Caesar salads I've tasted, and we were both in the mood. When we walked in, the hostess recognized us and took us back to a table. Watching the young attractive hostess and my wife as we were being led to our table made me thankful for the woman I married; she looked every bit as good as the young thing taking us to our table. We sat, and the waitperson came to take our drink order. As we gave our drink order, we heard a high-pitched scream practically in my ear. I turned around in my chair and found that we had been seated next to a family with a child and the child's chair backed up to my chair. If I hadn't been so interested in the way the two women walked on the way to be seated, I would have noticed the family and requested a different table. Before Surgery, I was fairly tolerant. After Surgery, my fuse is short. I felt for the parents of the child. After all, how can you train kids to be human in a restaurant if you don't take them to a restaurant? I just don't want to be part of the training ground. As the fingers started across the chalkboard again, excuse me, I mean the kid started to wail again, I looked at my wife and shrugged. I said to myself, "I can hold my breath longer than this kid can scream. It will be gone soon." This incident served to remind me that patience is not my long suit. I know it would not be correct for me to say something to the parents, but in my state of mind it took every ounce of restraint I could muster. I know the mom and dad of this cacophony were properly embarrassed, and I felt for them. That didn't stop me from wishing that the waitress would come by with one of those thirty-three gallon trash bags and place it over the howling kid. That would serve a dual purpose: not only would it mute the noise but it would also keep the mess to a minimum.

As a matter of fact, why not issue a bag at the door to every family with *younguns*? A bit like offering a lobster-bib for those who need it. This idea might be a good one for some of the adult diners, but I'm afraid it would dampen the repeat biz for the restaurateurs. I'm sure it would also cut the waitperson's tips down considerably. I'll keep working on this problem of crying babies. I'm sure there is a happy solution somewhere.

Fortunately, the family left before we were served our dinner. My wife knows screaming kids are not my favorite things under any circumstances. After the family was out of earshot, she said, "Did you enjoy the serenade?" She went on to say, "Dick, you have to learn to be more tolerant. The world is not going to do what you want; the world is going to do what the world does. It may not be any fun to have the child crying while you're trying to have a nice quiet dinner but that is the real world. You'd best come up with a strategy to handle that type of problem because you know that won't be the last time it happens."

Howling babies, yippee dogs and fingernails on the chalkboard all seem to have the same effect on me: they are just the wrong pitch or tone or something. I suppose I could go into meditation or do my mantra. Aqua, blue and white, aqua, blue and white: the aqua of the Caribbean, the blue of the sky as it touches the sea, and the white of the sand. But all that tends to take away from the pleasure of dining with my wife. I have to come up with a strategy to beat this little phobia of having howling babies, yippee little dogs, and fingernails on the chalk board. It is crazy and shows lack of control to let these things get to me. I'll beat it, I just have to figure out how.

There are lots of things in life you have to learn to have patience with. I've learned how to beat the long lines in grocery stores. It's nothing new, I just check out the front pages on the magazine rack. The covers seem to be made up mostly of the beautiful people and alien abduction.

Traffic is another area where you must have patience. I've got that whipped - I sing along with the golden oldies. These are things I can't control, so I have to learn how to live with them. Maybe I can use this philosophy with the crying babies. I should have just turned around and started singing to the kid. I don't know though; in today's society that may be considered molesting, and I would have to take the chance of having my singing bothering the rest of the patrons worse than the baby's crying.

Going to a restaurant calls for patience, but if there is no crying kid at least you can people-watch while you're waiting for your waitperson. I have had the feeling in some eating establishments that the second coming of Christ is going to occur before the waitperson does. I've got to remember that I have to fit into the world. The world is not going to work around me.

How about *waiting* in any professional's office: doctors, lawyers or Indian chiefs? I use this time to catch up on my escape reading.

If your patience fuse is as short as mine is, establish strategies to overcome. Don't be as irritable as the howling little kid. Bring a book or a hobby and if all else fails count your toes. But for heavens sake, be in control.

Talking with fellow rehabbers, I have uncovered a major inequity. It seems that many of us feel that although we are brain-damaged, we expect the rest of the world not to be brain-damaged. Unfortunately, this is not realistic. Every person I know has symptoms. I hear things like:

- "Now why did I go upstairs? What was it I was going to do? I was going to add something on to the grocery list. What the heck was it?"
- "I know I know you. I just can't remember from where or what your name is."
- "What was the name of that tune again? We used to sing it all the time."

- "Did I take my morning meds?"

We rehabbers don't want to forget that you folks who support us and help us on a daily basis don't walk on water either. You are human and subject to the frailties of being human. We must be reminded that although we do the things mentioned above a lot more than your standard bear, our support team, the angels, our relatives and friends, *are* human and subject to making an error now and again.

I told my wife, "If you make too many of this type of mistake, I will ask you to join me at rehab Tuesdays and Thursdays." When a cognitively-okay person has a lapse in memory, it helps them understand our problem better. After all, walking a mile or two in the other person's moccasins will help establish empathy.

My wife was standing in front of her closet saying, "I have no idea what I'm going to wear today." I was very tempted to say, "See there, your decision tool is broken, you need help." If that were the case, most of the folks who go to work in the morning would be heading for Project ReEntry or a similar group.

Suffice it to say there is a line somewhere and when you cross it the people who love you will probably have you checked out. All of us should be aware of our friends and loved ones, how we all act, react and interact.

Generally, from a cognitively injured person's point of view, there is no objective mechanism to tell what has been lost. Was a particular incident just a senior moment, or is that type of malady happening frequently?

Patience is a learned thing. I must study on that and be patient while I'm learning.

VOCABULARY

At first, when I couldn't find the word I wanted, it was like a slow suffocation of the mind. I'm learning to breathe slowly and take it easy. It is not the end of the world because there is a better word to explain what I want to say and I can't find it. I'm learning to handle it and, I might say, picking up a few new words along the way.

When I am writing or talking I will think, "What is that word I want? I know it will describe exactly what I am trying to say." Sometimes I think of my vocabulary as being on many huge Wheels of Fortune with words on all the stops. I can reach these words easily because I have RAM (random access memory). I just reach in and grab it. While my memory and vocabulary are interacting with each other searching for the word or phrase I want, I get this whirring noise. Then I get this mental recording in my head that says, "Sorry we are unable to make that connection, please try again later."

You guessed it: frustration, flooding and depression take over the whole system. It's been so bad at times I want to check my driver's license to make sure it is still me in this human shell. I know the word I'm looking for; it used to be part of my everyday language. Where the devil is it?

BOOKS

I like Koontz and King for the goose bumps. I've become friends with Cussler's Dirk Pitt. I wait with anticipation for Clive to tell me about the latest adventure of how he saved the world or found an old artifact. Patricia Cornwell created Kay Scarpetta. She's my kind of heroine. I have a love for Sci-fis as well. I have read a good many of the classics: Heinlein, Clarke, Bradberry. The Dune series and the Rama series were a couple of my favorites.

One of my favorite quotes about writers reading classics comes from Stephen King. He was asked if he had read any of the classics; he said, "I've read most of Dean Koontz." This tells me you don't have to be a classic writer to be commercially successful. I do believe "The Stand" by King is a classic. As a writer I just want people to enjoy my writing and gain something by reading it. What is important and different After Surgery, as opposed to Before Surgery, is I now get panicky if I don't have three or four books waiting to be read. Denny calls it my reading backup. She tells people that if I don't have a couple of books backed up, I go into reading withdrawal, and it is a terrible thing to see. I writhe on the floor and foam at the mouth. I never thought it was that bad, but I guess bad is in the eye of the beholder, like beauty, whether it be books or withdrawal.

By my choice, not a day goes by without some escape reading. I actually get hungry to read. It is just like I have missed two or three meals. Thank goodness I feel the same way about writing. If something happens that I don't write for a couple of days, it is a form of flooding to me. I have all these pent-up ideas and I must get them out or I will burst. I carry a pad and paper with me at all times to write down ideas, but that isn't enough. I must get them on my computer.

I don't know where the term *writer's block* comes from, but I sure don't have it. I always have ideas for new projects, follow-on books, new characters that I want to develop, and one of my favorites is *what-if ideas*. 'What if a flying saucer lands on your nose,' and then I'll take it from there. If you believe in reincarnation or past lives, I must have been an adventurer who kept a log. Even though my first book was a fantasy, I'm having a lot of fun doing this book. It is fun for me and cathartic, but I'm hoping it will be fun for the reader as well.

I hope that some of my mistakes will help others to not make the same ones, although that is rarely the case. It seems we human beings always want to create our own history. This means we will make our own mistakes and, hopefully, learn from them. Thank God I can read and write. It is enlightening to see someone else's mental creations. It is also thought-provoking for me to see what happens when I get a little creative myself.

TEXAN

I was born and raised in Madison, Wisconsin and proud of it. I had good times and good friends there, some I'm still in touch with. However, I do consider myself a Texan. I had put in a couple of stints in Texas doing different things at different times. The folks in Texas helped me get my doctorate in survival on several occasions. I've worked in Texas as a bellhop, poolroom cleaner-upper, gas station jockey, longshoreman, federal agent, national government sales manager of a large manufacturing company as well as several flavors of high-tech sales.

In all cases, the people of Texas have impressed me as being helpful, proud and loyal friends. I don't much care for some of the clichés about that, such as "I wasn't born in Texas, but I got here as quick as I could." Bullshit, I had my choice of living wherever I chose. I chose Texas and I'm proud to be a Texan. I was here in Houston before the boom years, through the boom years and after the boom years. I've been rich and poor in Texas and like most places, rich is better. Besides, Houston is only a few miles from the northern Caribbean — Galveston. The beaches may not be as pretty as Cancun, but the waters are healing and most folks have that laid-back attitude around the beach.

I will be a Texan till they cremate me and Denny pours my ashes into the Caribbean. So there!

Dr. See & TRC

When Denny realized the extent of my disability, she couldn't get anyone to listen to her. Everyone told her my brain was just fine.

Bless Dr. See, when we didn't know which way to turn, he knew. After talking to us for half an hour, he said, "You're right about that. Dick is not the same guy. He needs help. We need to see about getting him some rehabilitation. I suggest you talk to the Texas Rehabilitation Commission first. Then you need to be under the care of someone who understands endocrinology. I'll set an appointment with Doctor Michelle Zaniewski."

"Thank you," said my wife. "I was certain you would know how to help."

She turned and looked at me and said, "Honey, you are not able to do the things you used to do."

I looked at both of them and said, "We all know the man I used to be is gone." Lucky for us, we later realized that we get to create the new man. We agreed that we would work together to create the man we both wanted.

I finally got some guidance from the Texas Rehabilitation Commission (T.R.C.). They suggested I go to a place called Project ReEntry, where I would be tested, evaluated and then given a rehabilitation plan. I didn't know it then, but I was on my way to creating the new Dick Schmelzkopf.

Once I started the testing, I realized how bad a shape my brain was in. I actually felt embarrassed for doing so poorly on the tests.

MEDICATIONS

I got a little bonus when they went in to remove the tumor from my pituitary gland. What they didn't cut out, they disconnected. That makes this a case of brain-damage AND hypopituitarism.

The pituitary is the master gland that tells the other glands what to do and when to do it. The thyroid won't work without it. My internal temperature control is broken and I don't produce testosterone anymore. I'm tired more than I'm not. My bad cholesterol is leaping disproportionately over my good stuff. So I'm doing levoxyl, cortisone, baycol, hGH Nutropin, (human growth hormone). This is a needle a day. It goes on the same list as brushing my teeth, and combing my hair. I do it every morning and probably will for the rest of my life, and thank God it's available.

Then there is the testosterone. Due to the pituitary damage, my body is unable to manufacture testosterone which causes the inability to have an erection. I give myself a shot every three weeks in the hip. Testosterone has the same viscosity as syrup, so when I'm filling the syringe, I get some extra time to think about how great it is to be able to make love to my wife. I give my shot just above and to the right of my crack. I can't see what I'm doing, but I've gotten to where I can feel how everything is going. The needle is about the size of a railroad spike (or so it seems when I stick myself). But for all the complaining, I love the results and so does Denny.

My wife is a strong believer in alternative medicine. She has me on ten or twelve other types of stuff like ginkgo, green tea, garlic, saw palmetto, to name a few. With no pituitary, my immune system doesn't work very well. On the other hand, I have been healthy for the last few years. It is a pain to take all the meds, but as my dear departed father-in-law Captain George Washington Davis, the Fifth, USN Retired, used to say, "It is much better than the alternative."

He is right; death is so permanent and I have many more books to write, lots more people to help, and an untold number of Caribbean beaches to walk. Not to mention all the dark beers and piña coladas I have yet to taste. So I take my medication like I'm supposed to. For anybody who might have plans to take any of my advice, follow my lead on the medication thing (not necessarily my lead on the steak and spirits ideas).

Dr. Z, Endocrinologist

I've never been a big eater, but I enjoy the ceremony. When my wife and I are in the islands, I love to sit with her, get into each other's minds, and explore, while we are eating, the things we want to start when we hit the lottery and chat about which way we want to walk on the beach. We make the whole ritual of eating fun, from when we decide which restaurant we will enjoy for that meal, down to the dessert, then we head for where the Caribbean touches the sand.

Not everyone knows it, but when you walk with the person you love and have the Caribbean water washing up on your ankles, there is no greater mental release—no greater stress, frustration, or flooding antidote. The water washes up on my ankles and washes away all the negative stuff that has occurred since the last time I walked these waters.

Eating, ah yes. A change in my eating habits. I have always been fond of eggs, in any fashion, but my reaction to egg shell in my food is new. Not that anybody likes egg shell in their food, but I have almost a violent response to biting into a piece of shell. To me, now, crunching on an egg shell is the equivalent to *scraaaping* a fingernail on the chalkboard. I find now that I am much more persnickety about having one food run into another on my plate. God forbid that my peas should touch my mashed potatoes. Who knows what type of contamination could take place?

Dr. Z told me that I have to watch my cholesterol. I need to be particularly careful because I have no pituitary gland. This gland helps regulate that type of stuff. I watched my diet very closely for the first three months and eating became a chore rather than a pleasure. I looked back on my first cogent thought after surgery, which was be concerned about "quality of life." Fortunately Dr. Z got me into an experimental plan at MD Anderson Cancer Center, where Dr. Friend is doing testing on people with no pituitary gland.

With this test I need to inject HGH (human growth hormone) daily. This seems to help in keeping my bad cholesterol within acceptable range. Thank goodness, because I have made up my mind that I am going to watch cholesterol from a distance from now on. This is where I bring my ace-in-the-hole into play. Always remember *Quality of life*. My "Quality of life" calls for steak when I want it, as well as a little glass of spirits when I have the urge, much to the chagrin of my endocrinologist.

I am very fond of the Outback Steak House. The owner even has a method for cooking steak called "Dick's Way". Some people call it Pittsburgh; I rather like "Dick's Way," burnt on the outside and medium rare in the middle.

EDUCATION

I wasn't sure what kind of help I should be getting to become a writer. Should I take a basic English course or what? People have asked me what kind of education I have. I told them I am a road scholar (not to be confused with Cecil Rhodes' endeavor, when he set up an educational grant to Oxford for the very talented.)

I gained my doctorate in survival by bumming around the world for a decade. I specialized in survival under any circumstances. Pieces of my doctorate were gained in the United States; I've worked in every state accept Alaska and Hawaii and part of my doctorate was earned in foreign countries.

I mean, after all, how can you say you have a degree in higher learning without having some worldly experience? So I picked up some of the necessary credits by living in, visiting, or working in such countries as Canada, I panned for gold in British Columbia and fished in several other provinces. Mexico—I was a U.S. federal agent for four days.

There is another story. I smuggled tequila and rum into the U.S. (that was the era of the orange cowboy boots and sombrero). I always thought it was my personal responsibility to make sure the economy of Mexico stayed healthy, so I drank as much *Dos Equis* amber and *Negro Modelo* as I could possibly hold at any one time, as well as. . . as many times as I could. Now I find that I don't ingest quite as much as I used to, but I am enjoying it more. Better balance and better eyesight with a smaller investment.

Back on track, I can include Italy, Sicily, Germany, Libya, Lebanon and I stopped overnight in Panama to sample some of the different wares on my way to Australia. I did a great deal of graduate work in Sydney—incredible place with unbelievably kind people. I worked my way to Australia as a third cook on a German freighter called the *Cap Villano*. Before we got off the ship, another Yank, two Aussies and I were cited for mutiny. I think there may be a story in there, what do you think? I planned on being a bridge painter when I got to Sydney, but I was told that type of work paid minimum wages down under, so I got my first real selling job.

Since receiving my doctorate in survival, I have been doing post graduate research in the Caribbean. I'm going to continue my work in the Caribbean Islands till I get my doctorate in piña colada. As long as I'm there, I think I will go for at least a masters in local Island beers. *Red Stripe* from Jamaica and *Polar* from Aruba are nice, but so far nothing beats Mexico's *Negro Modelo* and *Dos Equis*.

So much for education. I just wanted you to know I have not neglected my mind. It was mostly fun picking up my D I S U A C Doctorate in Survival under any condition. May be my next book!

TESTING

I was given well over fifty tests to determine what was and was not working in my brain.

In what areas do I need support and reinforcement?

What is the best way for me to learn how to cope?

What method should the rehab people take to get me to get new synapses snapping?

The old me is gone. How do we get the new me as cognitively capable as possible? I won't bore you with all the little tests, but I wanted you to have a feel for how thoroughly these people examined me—numerous tests for sight and hearing to make sure I didn't have that type of challenge as well as a cognitive problem. I do, but they are minimal.

Project ReEntry defines *cognitive* as "the means by which we become aware through thought and perception." This includes reasoning, judging, thinking, conceiving, and remembering. These are the *executive function skills*. As it turns out, these are the areas that were in the little notch they cut out of my gray matter. I guess that's why I'm in cognitive rehabilitation.

Brain Damage

Since working with the people at *Project ReEntry*, I am aware that one of the things that is chiseled in cement is:

"There is a lot of gray area when you are working with your gray matter."

This may not be a brilliant perception, but I find alot of answers are like *not necessarily so, most of the time, as a general rule, under certain conditions that might be true.* Getting the answer to some questions is like trying to capture a spot of mercury the size of a dime under your thumb:

How long will I be in rehabilitation?

Will my memory ever be as good as it used to be?

These show me there are some questions that just don't have black and white answers. If I'm smart, I'll be in rehab for the rest of my life. I've got some new pathways working, and I'll get a lot more working before it's all over. I will learn new things every day. Nothing gets new pathways going faster than new stuff.

TEST RESULTS

*T*he findings from the tests I took erased all doubt about how much I had lost during my surgery and recovery.

I still wanted to be in denial about losing some gray matter capabilities. No denial now!

"These are the facts mam, just the facts."

My deficits fall mainly under the area of executive skill functions: impulsivity, cognitive inflexibility, memory for procedures, frustration control, visual scanning, and problem solving. How's that for a dirty laundry list? Not to worry, a mere bagatelle for a stepper like me. This is where it all began. You can't fix it unless you know what is broken. Now that we all know what ain't working, Project ReEntry gave me a strategies plan. The plan is nine pages long, and in great detail. The object is to get me back into polite society, whatever that means to me.

Some of the areas I will work on for the rest of my life are things like verbal memories, meaningful or logical memory, and memory for procedures. This one has been particularly difficult for me. Pattern recognition and note-taking also fall into this area. My cursive handwriting looks more like you asked a five year old to draw what a can of worms spilled on a paper would look like. I am now printing everything except my signature, which is also an interesting piece of work.

My wife said that if I could get a letter to Santa, and if he could read it, he would be sure to give me what I wanted. That would be after telling the elves, "This poor kid needs help. Get him a tutor for his penmanship, we'll teach him to spell at the same time."

The strategies go on and on. Visual memory, attention to detail, more attention to detail. This is a biggie for people with my kind of deficit. Information processing—I found that it is possible to drive someone crazy asking questions, especially if you ask the same questions over and over and over again. I don't know how the counselors keep sane.

We study verbal expression. This too can get old. I find that if someone asks me, "What time is it?" I tell them how to build a clock. As a Yiddish grandmother might say, "Along with being brain-damaged, you also have schill-schull (diarrhea in Yiddish) of the mouth. Hyperfluency—that means I'm talking too fast. If I am talking too fast, I am engaging my mouth before I engage my brain, absolutely guaranteed to get me in trouble whether I am brain-damaged or not.

"Presentation" means writing down notes and giving some type of talk on them. It makes no difference what the subject is. I have no aversion to speaking to a crowd, so that part doesn't bother me but staying on track seems rather difficult. My first experience for my listeners was probably a little like eavesdropping on my talking to Jonathan Winters and Robin Williams about dieting, and they are talking to me about the advantages of giving double-talk to their psychiatrist. It may not have made a lot of sense to the listeners, but they did laugh a couple of times and I did get better (discounting the reindeer fiasco - another story).

I worked on visual discrimination. Insight is high on the list of things to do. Two things they say to use as strategies are quite challenging. The first is: KEEP AN OPEN MIND. I'm all for that. B S (Before Surgery) having an open mind was very important to me. A S (After Surgery) however, is a different story. I have proven to myself time and again just exactly what cognitively inflexible means. Take copious notes—that's all well and good. I must draw each letter of my printing, which is very, very slow and still does not guarantee I will be able to read it.

If I write slowly, I may forget my thought; if I write fast, I can't read my notes. But that's as it should be: if it were easy, we would have no brain-injured folks. So we all work very hard on our individual treatment plans. *Initiation*, for a reason I don't yet understand, is that we find it hard to start something. It's just true. Initiating different projects is a good practice for this deficit.

Many, many projects and tasks have been accomplished by goal setting. I've been a goal setter for a long time, so that part is not so tough. My problem was where do I want to start. Until you know what you want to be or do, how do you set a goal? A goal is a map to help you reach that conclusion, whatever that may be. When you don't understand the conclusion, it's tough.

Second is planning: I plan my day. When am I going to do what task? Most of the time it works very well. Plan your work, and work your plan. No magic there. Unless of course you get buried in one of the tasks. I got into a computer game called *Bulldozer* which is mostly a plan ahead game. I would find myself getting behind in the schedule. This would cause me to get frustrated; after all I'm falling behind on my goal to do all these tasks. The counselors would remind me that **this** is **my** game; if I need more time, write it into the rules. I like writing my own rules. We as people don't take enough time and effort to rewrite much of the junk that is inundating our world. We might start by writing a rule that says whenever we meet someone on the street we have to give them a smile and say howdy.

Impulsivity is a detriment to the executive function area, so they tell me. I don't know about that. That is one of the things I used to like about myself. I would do a lot of things for instant gratification. Such as when I decided to bum my way to Australia on a German freighter, I made up my mind in about five minutes. Our basic learning is in the area of managing anxiety, stress, and frustration. These plague us all. I might add fear to this list. Unfortunately, all of these maladies feed on each other. If you let that get to you, you can count on it all turning into a ball of goo that gets bigger and bigger.

I know something about brain-damaged people, if my memory serves me and it is not a phantom memory. I also know about not being brain-damaged. Not being brain-damaged is better. But, I am creating the new Dick. I have to. If there is something about myself I don't like, I will change it, maybe to an attribute of a person I admire and like. I will be the type of person I would like to hang around with. I will have a positive attitude and the desire to do new and exciting things. And with a little more hair, if it won't ruin the grand scheme of things.

ANGELS AT REHAB

My first counselor, Donna, was a tall pretty lady from Jamaica. She was the person who very patiently helped me learn the ropes at Project ReEntry. She was always there to give me a helping hand, or some positive reinforcement, or whatever she felt I needed at the moment. We would swap stories about her beloved Jamaica. She influenced me on a children's story I wanted to write about twin reindeer from the Caribbean, called the "The Blue-Nosed Reindeer of the Caribbean."

Michael, another angel, was most influential in helping me understand the pitfalls of run-on and incomplete sentences. He had the patience of Job.

Glenda is the good angel of the west. She is always there to help out, especially with the frustration.

Tommy Tech bailed me out of computer frustration more times than I can count. I came very close to eating a couple of the computers, or at bare minimum, throwing one or two up against the wall.

Zen Master Lisa showed me how to manage frustration through meditation.

These angels and more helped me create the new Dick. I'll do my best to make you all proud.

First Day At Project Re-entry

I was feeling sorry for myself when I walked into the general assembly room. However, after talking and interacting with some of my fellow rehabbers, an old proverb came to mind, "I felt sorry for myself because I had no shoes, till I met the man who had no feet." When I looked around to see what kind of shape the rest of these people were in, I felt ashamed for being so self-centered.

I think Norman Vincent Peale had me in mind and was trying to give me some direction when he made this statement:

"The secret of life isn't what happens to you, but what you do with what happens to you."

Amen, brother. I'll beat this thing, then turn it into a friend. After a few years of wallowing in pity, I realized that I had better change my attitude.

One young lady in her early twenties suffers from cognitive impairment, thanks to a drunken driver. She has a tough time getting it together, never mind carrying it. She didn't say this, but after talking to her and watching her, I think she very well could have:

"Sometimes I stop to think and forget to start again."

One of the old sayings that people use when they are describing a large task to be done and how to start it is "How do you eat an elephant?"

"One bite at a time."

Meeting some of my fellow rehabbers and comparing the areas that I need to work on versus the areas they have to work on introduced me to humbleness. Each of us has his own trials and tribulations to face. All of our deficit areas make up each of our own elephants. If we each eat our own elephants one bite at a time, I don't even have a snack next to some of the other elephants I've seen up there.

Each morning they open the doors promptly at nine. A schedule is always posted pairing a rehabber with an angel and our names are posted on the bulletin board with a list of tasks that we are to work on for that day. These tasks are designed to strengthen each of our deficit areas. The assignments will help us get back into social life, the work arena or just get us back intermingling with regular folks without falling on our faces and embarrassing ourselves as well as the people we are trying to mingle with. We may also pick tasks ourselves to help us strengthen any areas that we would like to improve on our own. There is no end to the different puzzles, scenarios and situations that can be offered, as well as many flavors of computer work. I will go into a couple of the tasks, to give you an idea of the building that we need to do.

Out of the list of tasks that was under my name I chose to go for the mail office scenario. They put me over in a corner with a six inch stack of postcards and a pigeonhole for each of twenty states. The object is to put the right zip code in the proper pigeonhole. This task is very procedural. As you know by now, procedures are tough for me. The counselors told us,

"Don't get too frustrated; take a break if you need to."

The angels may have two or three rehabbers at a time. If I sat back and watched the angels, I noticed they kind of floated from one rehabber to another. Like good specters, they would hover for an extra moment with those who needed some help or a little extra attention. At first I couldn't figure out why I was doing a particular job. What was I trying to improve with this task, procedure, or what have you? So I asked. It was a matter of memory and procedures. I ended up taking several breaks.

We have several types of group meetings. In the health group we talk about good mental health, like keeping a good attitude. We also talk about the values of good hygiene. We do not take the road Tom Lehrer talked about:

"Clean mind, clean body, take your pick."

We work on total health, inside and out. In today's world we would say "Keep your keyboard clean and make sure you're using the right software." Trying to figure out if we are using the right software was the difficult part. The whole thing translates to bathe, brush your teeth, and have a good attitude. And for crying out loud, keep a smile on your face. Some of us have more to smile about than others.

We also have a group called STAR. In this group we practice situations and job interviews. We may tape them for critiquing or for ideas on how we might improve. One day I was acting the part of the human resource person interviewing a secretary. This scene could be very typical. A sister rehabber came in, shook my hand and said, "I'll do a better job for you than somebody without a handicap. When can I start?"

Maybe not the best interviewing style but she sure got my

attention. This type of attitude is just what rehab is all about. I wanted to encourage this type of thinking so I told her, "As of this moment you are on the payroll."

She lit up like Times Square. I was proud of her and I was proud of me for giving her a high for the day. When I am working with one of the people in worse shape than I am, I get to thinking I'm a counselor. At any rate, no harm done and a smile on the face of the person I helped. You know how good it feels to help someone? It almost always does me more good than it does them. This is the kind of feedback we rehabbers need. Unfortunately real life is not like this. People are reluctant to hire us, or, for that matter, to socialize with us.

If employers would check with the mayor's office, they would find a huge database from which to draw loyal personnel.

We had one session called *games*. We would play games for an hour. This session was good for showing us how to play well together in the sandbox. It is astonishing to me how we can get twenty people together who are known to get frustrated easily, have limited social skills, maximum depression, as well as frustration, no patience, and a fuse that could go off in a New York minute (in Texas, that's thirty-seven seconds). Yet we interact better than a party of diplomats, well, most of the time. We don't beat our shoes on the table or call each other names—not much, anyway.

If you watch the state of affairs in the world—the fighting and the starvation—or watch the news, it's there every night. We get along far better than most countries negotiating for peace. We actually get things resolved occasionally.

DAY TO DAY REHAB

I attend Project ReEntry every Tuesday and Thursday from 9:00 a.m. till 4:00 p.m. Every morning they have some type of test or task that will challenge me in one of my weaker areas. One problem they give us to solve is called Earth Tour. This is a real beauty. They supplied me with an atlas, an almanac, and thirty questions that went like this.

> From Egypt, swim across the _____ sea to Turkey, where 99% of the population is of the _____ religion. Next, hop a flight to Katmandu, in the country of _____ and travel by yak directly to the capital of India, named _____. India has many citizens (population) _____ and it is way too crowded for comfort. Rent a baby elephant to take you to the largest city in Thailand, called _____.

To find the solution to thirty of these questions I am bopping back and forth between the reference books like a yo-yo.

This kind of challenge makes me use many strategies, which of course is the name of the game.

There are lots of tests like *Which House Does the Zebra Live In?* These are deductive reasoning quizzes. The object is to get new synapses snapping, create new neural pathways to take the place of the ones that were damaged.

Sometimes when we all get to studying, the air even gets tense. The only things moving are the wheels in the rehabbers' heads. Some of us need to put a little grease on our wheels, but then again, that's why we are here. Sometimes everything is so quiet you could hear a mouse break wind.

It is not all labor. Here's one based on humor. It is called *Solving Riddles*. "What animal keeps the best time?" I didn't print the answer upside-down at the end of the book like Rehab does, but the answer is "a watchdog."

"What never asks any questions, but everyone answers it?"

"Telephone." Thirty pages of these.

Understanding word drawings tested my imagination as well as my deductive powers. This consists of a group of letters that represent a familiar word or phrase. Try these two and see what you get.

MIND
MATTER   PpOpD

How about Mind over matter and two peas in a pod?

This is one I missed.   E Z
                         iiiiiiiiiiiiiii
Easy on the Eyes.

There are hundreds of these. They sure do make a guy think. One more, to keep you on your toes.

DO ft OR.

Spelling tests, writing tests, vocabulary, definitions, synonyms, homonyms, circle the picture that is different, draw this pattern from another angle. Tests where you must follow the directions exactly, step by step, or you can't solve the problem. There are math tests, judgment and reasoning tests, and lots of different kinds of memory tests.

Lunch at rehab is from noon till one. I sometimes come back from lunch and do the pipe exercise. This is counting and categorizing PVC pipe pieces to an ordering form. My totals of each type will let me know what I need to order to keep my inventory at the level it must be maintained. This test convinces me I could never be a stocker and order stuff. I never had that much interest in knowing the difference between an elbow joint and a T-bar, as far as plastic pipe was concerned. The stocker thing would be about as much of a challenge to me as being a professional clock-winder. In a word, boring. It's like counting your toes over and over again; once I have established that I have ten of them, I think the fun is over. On the other hand, I should *inspect* what I *expect*, so I count them again.

My most favorite is a computer challenge where you push rocks around. There were fifty levels of competence on this test. I did all fifty, but the frustration factor was incredibly high. I came close to throwing the computer out the window several times but over a period of months I beat it. Never, never say die. As you can see I could go on and on with the tests. I just wanted to give you a flavor for rehab. Oh by the way, **DO ft OR** is a foot in the door.

When I started studying areas of cognitive deficit and trying to improve my weak areas, I found it amazing how much I had lost. As an example, I used to have a very good vocabulary. Now when I reach for a word I want, my mental motors just keep grinding on, not stopping at the correct word. It is alot like thumbing through a book and not finding the place I wanted to stop. Then I find myself checking the Thesaurus quite frequently, but that's okay, this is just another strategy to help me improve my present state. My spelling has never been great, but with the advent of the computer and Spell-check, I'm as good as the next guy.

My first day in Project ReEntry for cognitive rehabilitation we had an introductory meeting. This is where everybody introduced themselves and told how long they had been coming here, what they expected to gain by participating in this ordeal and how they got there. Again, "I felt bad because I had no shoes, till I met the man who had no feet." Believe me when I say "Shame on me for being such a cry baby." Several of the rehabbers needed physical rehabilitation as well as cognitive rehabbing. Donald, who is the center of one of my favorite stories, has been in a wheelchair for a number of years due to an auto accident. He has partial use of one of his legs. The angels talked him into trying to walk with a walker and braces. The first few times he tried, he had everybody teary-eyed. It is a magical thing to watch a man who hasn't walked for years trying to get back on his feet. An angel would walk behind him, just in case. On occasion, he would fall down. We would all gasp. He would crawl over to a desk or something stable and climb back up.

You talk about inspirational! He has left us now because of government funding, or I should say, the lack of it. But I know he is out there somewhere, trying his best. I used to kid him about making the four-minute mile. I'll tell you, don't be surprised. He has the will and a positive attitude, and as we say, "Never, never give up."

A couple of our members couldn't speak coherently. A couple of them couldn't remember the names of the counselors, even though they have been going to rehab every day for two or three years, working with the same people.

Most had disaster stories to tell about their mates. *Ninety percent* of the rehab participants had lost their Significant Other because the Other could not stand to be around them or couldn't take the added responsibility of helping that person find strategies to aid them to overcome the mental problems. *Fifty percent* had severed ties with their family and friends.

We talk frequently about how fortunate we are, Denny and I. It is so important to have support at home, as well as friends and relatives who stick by you through such a difficult ordeal. The horror stories I heard were enough to make me cry when I was alone and thinking about all the rehabbers that were trying to fit back into the system after having the system stick it to them. These were the people who worked hard all their lives to be fine, upstanding citizens, contributors to society. These are the real people who keep this world going. These are people whose companies threw them out because they couldn't do what they used to do. They had wives or husbands who took all the money and left.

Rehabbers would talk about friends who never returned phone calls. It doesn't take long to find out who is still loyal to you as a friend and who the fair weather friends are. Thank God most of my friends saw my problem and were anxious to help me in any way they could. Relatives didn't seem to be bothered by the fact that I was a new person, at least I was trying to create the new Dick. I have always been something of a rebel. I guess they figured this was just another part of me. Love him or leave him.

The love has been overwhelming. Denny, the love of my life for thirty years now, took it all in stride. She realized that the old Dick was gone and she was going to help me create the new one. I am told by Russ and Dr. Pollock, my number one angel, that they think she is doing a grand job in helping me build the new me.

I Finally Stopped Drooling in Public
or
I Know Who I Used to Be, But Who Am I Now?

*W*hat was that again? This was the title of the book until the publisher got hold of it. Now it is only a chapter title.

I got the idea of "I Know Who I Used To Be, But Who Am I Now?" when I first started writing my fantasy book. I was thinking, "What would my rehab story be called?" This says it all. I could remember the successful high tech sales guy, I just couldn't do it any more. At that point I wasn't sure what I was or what I wanted to be. Thus, "But Who Am I Now?"

Denny tells me when I first came home from the hospital I drooled a bit. Then I would make that slurping sound to stop drooling "Most irritating," she said. So I used to kid our friends and say, "I stopped drooling in public so Denny can take me out now. Sh*lurrrp.*"

My publisher, Chris, bless his heart, said, "If you want this book to be found by people who can really use it, you have to have the problem in the title." That's why we discussed adding pituitary dysfunction to the title. Certainly these things are all tied together. Why treat the pituitary problem like it was a red-headed step-child? After all, folks with a pituitary problem need help, too. If the person who has a pituitary dysfunction got it the same way I did, he/she probably has the same deficits. It might be a long title, but it makes sense to me. Is that good or bad when it makes sense to someone who is cognitively-challenged?

Bob, my pool-playing buddy, was at the house and I was telling him what my publisher was saying relative to who was going to read this book.

Bob said, "You need something snappy for a title. If you have both a pituitary dysfunction and brain-damage, what do you think of this as a title "Dueling Drooling"? Or how about this, "Brain-damaged, Pituitary, Drooling & Me."

I said, "Let's see what the publisher has to say. He is the expert so I think I'll let him have the last word."

During this conversation Bob made the comment that, on the rare time that I win playing pool, it's his loss. He says he writes off the mileage from his house to my house as well as the loss at the pool game. He calls it a donation to the cognitively-challenged. I'm not sure what the IRS would think about that, but we both had a good laugh out of it. Good old Bob, always thinking. I told him if that's the way he writes off his pool losses, I should write mine off as therapy or maybe ongoing education. In fact, this is really an addition to my doctorate in survival. In the process of getting my doctorate, I do pick up the price of a beer now and then.

WHO'S BRAIN-DAMAGED?

The angels encourage us to take breaks if we get frustrated. A fellow rehabber and I were taking a smoke break and when we got outside to the smoking area, we noticed a guy from the building changing a tire in the hot Texas sun. We had seen him around our floor as a nodding acquaintance; he was a physical therapist whose office was on the same level as Project ReEntry. He was just getting the last lug nut off the wheel and putting it in the hubcap beside him. As he stood to wipe his brow he acknowledged us with a nod and a "Boy, it's a hot one today." He wasn't paying any attention to what he was doing and he kicked the hubcap. All the lug nuts promptly went down a storm drain. He said looking at us, "Well, isn't *that* dandy? Now what am I going to do?"

He kicked the tire and cursed. I walked over to him and said, "Why don't you take one nut from each wheel and put it on this one. Then you can head for a dealership, service station or parts store, replace your missing lugs and you're in business again."

He said, "That's a great idea. I thought all you guys at Project ReEntry were brain-damaged." I looked at him and his situation, then I looked at my rehab buddy, gave him a wink, and then looked back to the guy with the tire problem.

I said to myself, "I can't resist it." I looked him in the eye and said, "We're brain-damaged, but we're not stupid." Then I set about helping him. My partner came off the smoking bench and offered help, too.

The physical therapist said, "My apologies, guys. That was my ignorance showing. I know better, I see you people working every day. My mouth started running before my mind was engaged."

My rehabber buddy says, "You would be amazed at how much of that is going around. Because we think a little slower sometimes doesn't mean we don't think."

I couldn't have said it better. I added in a kind way, "They removed a brain tumor—they didn't give me a lobotomy."

I've watched the PT guy on several occasions. He never passes one of us without saying "Howdy." I made a point of telling him thank you. "There are some folks up here who only get a greeting inside that door. It all helps to make a good day for you and us."

AWARENESS & BEAUTY

I guess I must be getting cross-compensated (like a blind person, in some respects). Even though I've got a small piece of gray-matter that doesn't seem to work like everybody else's, I believe my eye for color and movement is becoming more acute.

I was waiting in the van while Denny was doing some shopping when a bird flew into my peripheral vision and my eye caught it immediately. The bird dipped down and flew over a small bed of flowers. The colors struck me, so I stayed and looked at the flowers. There were some orange and some yellow. I find myself looking for beauty, whether it be birds, flowers, men or women. I do seem to notice the pretty ladies more than I used to, so Denny tells me. I wouldn't argue with that. I find myself paying more attention to blouses, shirts or ties, checking them over for color and design. I have sworn off ties. I can't imagine a situation that would call for me to wear a tie. That would include weddings, funerals, and awards. I see this as a form of freedom, most certainly not disrespect. (Of course, it might be something to do with not remembering how to tie one.)

When I see a brilliant color, I can almost taste it. This seems to happen more with flowers, birds and fish than anything else. I love it, I'll say to Denny when we are driving along in the spring, "Look at those bluebells and Indian paintbrushes, I can almost taste the gorgeous blue and the brilliant orange." Life is good at a time like that.

A WRITER

*I*n my mind, there are several steps to knowing where you are in the learning process.

There is *unconscious incompetence*—where you don't know what you don't know. How do you know what to study if you don't know?

Then there is *conscious incompetence*—where you know what you don't know. So you know what to study.

Unconscious competence—when you know it, but you don't know you know it.

My favorite, of course, is *conscious competence*—you know that you know. Very few people, in my opinion, reach this stage, but many people think they have.

Thanks to Guida I believe I have reached the point of conscious incompetence. I know I need to read, study and do everything I can do relating to creative writing. Someday, maybe I'll be able to teach. The people who say, "Those who can, do; those who can't, teach" are full of prunes. There is nothing that says you can't do both if you are so inclined. One of the greatest feelings is helping people help themselves. If you don't believe me, ask my guru, Dr. Guida Jackson, how she feels when one of her students wins an award or gets published.

It took me well over a year of rehabilitation to decide who the new me was going to be. When I started, I flat had no idea at all. Then I decided the new me was going to be a fiction writer. The process of writing a book allows me to employ strategies that will help me get new pathways in my brain working. The planning of plots and subplots, as well as character building and making sure that I don't have any incongruities helped me build my cognitive skills. I found the whole process very challenging and interesting. This will help get new synapses snapping. When I started studying my areas of cognitive deficit, trying to improve my weak areas, I found it amazing how much I had lost.

All I really wanted to be was a storyteller. If you want to have someone read your stories other than your friends and relatives, you have to be published. In order to be published, you must follow certain rules. These involve such things as point of view of the story, tense and person (who is telling the story). I decided as long as I was going to be a writer, I might just as well get published. This meant going to college. Going to college meant mingling in polite society with folks who didn't know about my brain damage.

After some investigating I found that Montgomery College in Montgomery, Texas would suit my needs. My first day in class was interesting. Our professor was a published author, Dr. Guida Jackson. Our class included a combination of writers and would-be writers. We were asked to introduce ourselves and tell what our reason was for taking the class. When it was my turn I stood, told them who I was, and that writing this fantasy book about wizards, witches and dragons was therapy for me, that I was cognitively-challenged, and as long as I was going to write, I might just as well get published. I spoke reasonably well, so it didn't seem to have an impact on the members of the class. Later they found out what I meant.

Typically we would write eight pages of our story at home. Then we would come to class and Doctor Jackson would lecture us on a fine point of creative writing. Next, one of us would pass around copies of our eight pages that we had done at home. The author would read his stuff and the others would correct, edit and make notes for ideas to the author on all sorts of things, like grammar, punctuation, choice of words, additional plot or subplot ideas. Then we would go over their writing word for word and make our suggestions and discuss the ideas, why they were good or not so good.

Though this process of reading aloud was very time consuming, it was also incredibly valuable to all of us. When I read my story with incomplete and run-on sentences included, my fellow classmates realized what I meant when I said cognitively-challenged. It took us twice as long to do my editing and critiquing as it did to do anyone else's. Bless their hearts, no one complained. Everyone helped me. I had a particularly hard time with point of view and staying in the proper person with the proper tense.

My creative writing had its pitfalls as well. I was having trouble writing a proper sentence; most sentences seemed to be incomplete or run-on. The frustration of having to rewrite and rewrite, and the depression of not being quite able to put it the way I wanted it was enough to make my buns grow together. I'm still working very hard to fix this problem. Thanks to Michael, the Golden Angel, the fix is coming along—ever so slowly, but moving in the right direction.

For sure, I'm no Shakespeare; however, there is perhaps no one who enjoys writing more than I do. Lucky for me, I have my own Web Page Master, Don. The only way to describe Don is to quote Ella May Morris, "He's a long tall Texan." Both Don and Donna, *Donner* as Don calls his wife, are tall enough that they look down on six footers, and when they say "Howdy, ya'll," it comes from deep in the heart of Texas. They are like most Texans I know, real people.

Bless his heart. He put together a web page for me with dragons and all. Dragons are a thing with me since I am writing a fantasy about them. He put several short stories on my web page. One about my dart buddies, I call it *The Intergalactic Playoffs* with Damon Runyan-type characters who parallel several darters in the league. It was challenging and fun to do this. It is an on-going Sci-fi saga.

Maybe I can get my fantasy published now that my story is out.

BOURBON

When I was in high school, one of the ways I made money was being a gas pump jockey. I worked at one of those stations that gave gifts: get ten gallons of gas and get a shot glass, or your first piece of peach luster dinnerware. I was happy to work on Christmas Eve; they were paying double time. One of the married guys got stuck as well. I felt for him; he was a newly married man with his first kid. I was only seventeen so it was against company policy for me to work the night shift alone.

It was December 24th, about eight in the evening, snowing like crazy, Christmas card picture-perfect, cold white and lots more coming down.

My partner for the night asked if I was a drinking man. I said sure; he left for the drug store two blocks away. He didn't know, and I never gave it a thought, but I had never had hard liquor before. I thought to myself, that's okay, I can hold a six-pack (and I might add, not very well). When Jim came back he asked me to go out to the showcase and bring in a couple of shot glasses. I did.

The traffic was practically non-existent. We went into the back room and he poured bourbon out of a pint bottle. We picked up the shots, clicked glasses, said Merry Christmas and threw the shot back. This was my first shot of bourbon; strangely enough it went down with no problem at all.

As he was running out the door he yelled back at me, "Pour us another shot, I got this one."

In the time it took him to gas and check under the hood, I filled his shot glass and drank the remainder of the pint of bourbon. My logic went like this: I'll buy the next one. After all, if I can drink a six-pack, I can certainly drink a pint.

When Jim came back in from the cold Wisconsin night, he went straight for the shot. He threw it back and, noticing the empty bottle he said, "Did you drink all that by yourself?"

"Sure, there's nobody here but me and the peach luster."

He said, "Are you used to drinking hard liquor?"

I said, "No, but I can hold a six-pack. Here's some more money, I'll watch the pumps while you get another bottle."

He said, "Fifteen minutes from now, you'll be so drunk you won't be able to find your ass with a search warrant."

Twenty minutes later I was outside looking at a sign that was ten feet high and twenty feet long. It was red, yellow and blue. I had seen this sign everyday for the last year but at that point I couldn't tell you what it said; for that matter, I couldn't tell what color it was. I remember waking up in the back room lying on the floor in a corner. My drinking partner had covered me with employees' jackets which were very nice, blue with fleece lining. I in turn had puked on the whole world, especially the jackets, and was about to do it again and again.

There are many things said about the classic hangover, but why did it have to be my first experience with bourbon? The next three days put me off drinking forever. At least that's what I told myself then. I didn't drink bourbon for twenty years.

At this time in my life, my usual mode of transportation was hitchhiking, but I was so sick I had to take buses. I couldn't imagine myself asking someone to stop so I could throw my guts out on the street. In taking a bus I never did make it from point "A" to point "B" without having to run up to the driver, get a transfer and ask him to let me off as soon as possible. They must have noticed I looked a little green around the gills, because the driver always stopped the bus right there and let me off.

There is no doubt in my mind that I had alcohol poisoning because my stomach informed me that everything I ate or drank had alcohol in it. It would throw it out of my body at a fierce rate, both from the top and the bottom (unfortunately, on occasion, both at the same time).

If I had it to do all over again (Please God, never again like that), I would have carried a barf-bag with me. Maybe it would have taken some of the urgency out of my problem, like a security blanket. It's not that I'd need it or might even use it; it would just be there.

A friend of mine once told me that, "Having diarrhea was the ability to shit through the eye of a needle at a hundred yards." If they ever decide to make that an Olympic event, I have been trained for the gold.

I got so I could *almost* control my puking through the heavy partying years. I would do well till the commode seat came down on the back of my head. I wonder if that could have had anything to do with… naw. I have learned from those episodes that some lessons are harder to learn than others.

You would think a bout like that would put me off the *demon liquor* forever. Ah, not so, my friend; I'm made of stouter material than that.

Excess alcohol and other strains to the system can cause death. I should know—I was at its door for three days. They wouldn't let me in; they said my breath would knock a buzzard off a garbage wagon. It certainly tasted like it would.

Be careful with self-medication.

ADD WONDERMENT TO BRAIN-DAMAGED

*I*s it because I'm brain-damaged and a writer that the English language seems challenging? Look at these examples of interesting English, most of them a wonderment to me:

- The bandage was wound around the wound.
- The farm was used to produce produce.
- The dump was so full it had to refuse more refuse.

> The "I" before "E" except after "C" rule can be interesting.
> It's a rule that is simple, concise and **efficeint.**
> For all **speceis** of spelling it's more than **sufficeint.**
> Against words wild and **weird,** it's one law that shines bright.
> Blazing out like a beacon upon a great **hieght.**
> In our work and our **liesure,** our homes and our schools,
> Let us follow our **consceince, sieze** proudly our rules!

> Will I dilute my standards, make them vaguer and blither?
> I say NO, I will not! I trust you will not **iether**.

I could go on and on with these, but I think this is enough to show you the consternation a new writer might go through or someone who has a doctorate in survival, not English.

Oxymorons also add some interest for the new writer or the alien trying to learn the language. I have many of these, but I wanted to mention a few to make a point.

act naturally
found missing
resident alien
clearly misunderstood
pretty ugly.

Like others, we have had our to-dos with the IRS, so I find this one of particular interest, *temporary tax increase.*

I have been trying to understand the English language for a good number of years. Like rehab, I'll keep working at it.

CECIL B. DEMILLE?
OR STEVEN SPIELBERG?

I came to Rehab on Tuesday at nine o'clock, standard procedure for me. I went directly to the bulletin board to see what challenges had been set out for me by the staff. They wanted me to work on my fantasy story. That's great, I thought, just what I had in mind. I found myself a vacant computer station and started writing. A few moments later Russ, the Assistant Director of this organization, came in and said, "Do you have a moment?"

Russ is not only a big wheel in the organization, he is also a big man with a big presence; there is no way not to notice this man. By the same token, there is no way I would not give him my complete time and attention when he speaks. He has bailed me out of computer problems time and time again. He also has an excellent sense of humor; when he gets my attention I never know if he is going to lay a joke on me or what. His joke telling is legendary. I gave him my full attention.

He continues, "We are expecting a large contingent of folks to come in Thursday for a conference on rehabilitation for the cognitively-challenged. There will be people from all walks of the rehab profession. That is, people who are interested in these matters. This includes doctors, lawyers and Indian chiefs. Dr. Pollock wants to give some type of presentation to them from the patient's point of view. Yesterday, we had a meeting of all the clients and they voted that you would be the best person to represent them and their point of view. Would you be willing to take this on as a project?"

I said, "That gives me today and tomorrow to put something together. Right?"

He nods his head and asks, "Are you sure you're up to it? I'm going to walk through the facility and take a video. We want you to do a voice-over—your choice on what you want to say and how you want to say it. We will run the video with the voice-over; if we like it, we'll keep it. If not, we'll run the video and I will explain what they are seeing. I don't think that would be nearly as interesting as what you could do."

That's Russ for ya. He is always good with a compliment and encouragement. How could I say no? I'm calling myself a writer; now is my chance to see if I can write on the fly, so to speak.

The possibilities were endless. How did I want to start this thing? After much deliberation, I decided a definition is the best place to start. After all Project ReEntry is a cognitive rehabilitation organization. What does *cognitive* mean? Cognitive means about the same whether you look it up in the medical books or the dictionary. Boiled down, its essence is this:

"*Cognitive: the means by which we become aware through*

> *thoughts and perceptions. This includes reasoning, judging, thinking, conceiving, and remembering."*

I wrote fifteen pages of dialog on this stuff, what this place means to me and the other clients. I made some before and after rehab comparisons. I talked about some of the strategies they teach us and how I have used them. I mentioned improvements I had seen in other rehabbers, the use of some of the tools offered here, and what they do for us. Dr. Pollock was kind enough to allow me to sit in on the session where they showed the tape with my voice-over. I got a standing ovation for my contribution. That sure did make me feel like a major contributor—and hey! I just might make it as a writer.

CREATIVITY

*W*ho knows where it comes from? Like many people before me have said, "If I could figure out how to put it in a jar, the world would be a better place." Creativity has struck me at odd times. I was coming back from rehab, the traffic was heavy, as always in Houston. Not being a great multi-tasking person, I was watching what was going on around me. It wouldn't hurt to be a seer driving in Houston traffic. I can see it now, I was driving along and saying to myself, don't change lanes, that little green car is going where I want to go. If that were the case and I could tell what was going to happen next, I could do a little heavier thinking while I was driving along. However that was not the case. A lightning bolt of a creative nature hit me. I thought of the wizard Zoltar in my fantasy book. The bolt was that I will have a twist to his magic portal for the next book. Zoltar creates a portal by taking something personal from someone. In the case of my current fantasy, it was a needle taken from the Duchess Nafair and then saying an incantation over a liquid, like wine or water, and finally dropping the personal item into the liquid. This allows the wizard to see everything that person is doing at the time they are doing it.

I visualize the wizard looking into the portal and seeing himself watching himself. Interspersed with flashes of the person he wanted to check on. When he sees the portal flash back and forth, he knows something is wrong.

I haven't decided if I want Zoltar to realize he has touched the personal object so that the portal sees him as well as the other person or if I want Illumina the witch to play a joke on him. I like the idea. I'll decide when I write the next book how to use it. I have a file for the different ideas that come to mind.

Meanwhile I have pulled over to the side of the road to write my ideas in my ever present note pad. I'm always afraid of micro-memory failure. I don't know how many ideas have been lost for not taking the time to write them down, but I know I have lost many.

If you have a problem as I do with multi-tasking and/or micro-memory failure, pull over to the side of the road and write your ideas down. Particularly if the pickup truck that is tailgating you has Texas tags and a gun rack. That's one truck you don't want to blend paint with.

READING TO LEARN

Most people want to learn new things (and if they don't, shame on them). We should all try to learn new things every day. When I read something to broaden my knowledge, it is a never-ending battle. The problem is, I may or may not retain it.

This applies to computer stuff, for example—getting online. I finally got to the point where I can receive and read e-mail, but I'm still having problems with the finer points. I haven't gotten the hang of doing attachments, or sending to multiple addresses, or sending something that I have received to someone else. When I receive a joke or information that someone I know would like, I have to make a copy and send in by snail mail.

This is a good time to talk about *pattern recognition*. My wife has set her screen so that it looks the same as mine. She asked me to turn her system on and get online. I couldn't figure out how to do it, even though both systems have the same icons. I'm working on it, and I know I'll get it eventually.

The road to the comfort level where it makes no difference what box I'm using seems to be bumpier than it should be. The box should be transparent to me. I need only to get online. Pattern recognition sucks when you have lost your executive functioning skills. Retention and retrieval are still major problems. I'll get it right if I have to work on it till judgment day.

Here's another pattern recognition problem: I have changed my wife's purse from the black one to the brown one dozens of times. I know where she keeps everything. Her purse is neat and orderly, always. She was cleaning eyeglasses one day and asked me to bring her all my glasses. Sunglasses, reading glasses, glasses for driving, the glasses I use for computer work.

Then she said, "Please get my glasses out of my brown purse." As soon as I located the purse, I looked through it and could not find them anywhere. I brought the purse to her and she opened the panel where she keeps them and, lo and behold, there they were, big as Dallas. (I say big as Dallas because the people in Dallas think they are bigger and better than Houston, when in fact, the only thing bigger is their heads.)

Well, back to the purse and the glasses. I even had my hand on them and I still didn't recognize them for what they were. Is this a *scotoma* (blind spot), or maybe a pattern recognition problem? Or just another joy of having a nick taken out of my gray matter? I find this lack of recognition gets in the way every now and again. Denny says it is a challenge with pattern recognition. The problem is similar to not getting the rack correct when playing pool.

NEGATIVITY, THE TERRIBLE TWOS & THE REBELLIOUS TEENS

Through this first two-year period my wife and I have had many strange experiences, including feeding myself, job hunting and adjusting to social life.

My wife tells me that period AS (After Surgery) was for her like raising a child. I went through the 'terrible twos'—anything new was automatically given a *no*. Denny would say, "Do you want to try this new restaurant?"

"No."

"Do you want to get that new shirt? It would really look good on you."

"No."

"Let's have some people over."

"No."

She tells me it didn't make any difference what she suggested: if it was new, the answer was no. She also tells me that during this period of the 'terrible twos,' I threw in a lot of the 'rebellious teens.' My darling bride tells me I went through, and for that matter, I'm still going through, a rebellious period. She might say "Why don't you get your hair cut?"

I would probably reply with something like, "Why? Who gives a hoot? I sure don't."

Just to lighten it up a bit, I'll share some of the things I did and thought when I first started to prepare my own meals. My skills in the kitchen have gotten better. Even so, making a peanut butter and jelly sandwich has its challenges. I couldn't remember what went on the bread first. A few times of trying to put butter on over the peanut butter, or butter on over the jelly, and I started getting the hang of it. This could be very messy, trying to put butter on top of your peanut butter and jelly. Making a grilled cheese had its bad times, too. "Do I put the pan on the stove first to get it ready for the sandwich?" A couple of times with the kitchen filled with smoke and my wife saying, "No Dick, get the sandwich ready first, *then* put it in the pan with the stove set on five." My strategies in the kitchen called for notes to remind me of the dangerous stuff, seeing that a mistake using the stove could be quite serious.

If I made a sandwich, I would leave drawers and cabinets open when I was finished and often leave the refrigerator door open or the stove on. My wife was smart enough to check on me whenever I tried a task on my own. She would say, "Did you mean to leave these things open?" It was amazing to me as I look back. Even walking around the kitchen fixing a sandwich, I couldn't tell there was anything wrong with open cabinets, drawers and all.

One night my wife shook me and said. "What are you doing?"

I was standing beside the bed urinating on our dresser. I thought I was in the bathroom. Max flooding! Humiliated, mad at myself, mad at God. How can I put my wife through this time and time again? Fortunately, this incident did not happen again. (At least, I don't think it did.)

FLOODING WHILE DRESSING

*F*or the first couple of years I wore nothing but snuggy-suits (sweatsuits) all day around the house. My wife would say, "We're going out for lunch." This might be at nine o'clock in the morning.

I would stand in front of my closet and say to myself, "Okay, she doesn't want me to wear blue jeans. I know, I'll wear my brown dress Wranglers with that blue shirt. Wait a minute, how about the blue shirt with that blue sport coat? Maybe I don't like those blues together. Okay, how about the gray coat, the black shirt and the black boots? I'm sure I'm not in the mood for those boots."

At twelve o'clock Denny would find me standing in front of my closet, unable to make a decision. She would have to say, "Don't worry about it, wear the blue shirt, the brown pants and the blue and brown sport coat with sneakers." If she hadn't helped me with what to wear, we wouldn't have got out of the house till the next season.

Even as I was standing there I realized I needed to make a decision, I would start flooding, and this just added to the frustration. Flooding and depression are like watching a huge snake devour itself. It goes on and on and on. A good thing has come out of this brain 'to-do': I don't have to worry about flooding while I'm trying to match my shirt, suit and tie. I no longer wear a suit or tie. Not to weddings, not funerals, nor *nothin'*.

When I tell this particular story my wife says that as far as dressing goes I was brain-damaged a long time ago. While I was getting my doctorate in survival, some thirty years ago, I was driving a truck in Texas when I got word that a buddy of mine was getting married in Washington, DC. He wanted me to be his best man. Well, I couldn't pass that up.

Another bumming buddy and I went to Del Rio and crossed the bridge into Boys Town, Mexico. After a rather raucous day and night doing the things you do in Boys Town, Larry and I filled the trunk with tequila and rum. We headed east for DC so I could be best man at the other buddy's wedding. I got the tux and all the trimmings. The family he was marrying into was quite conservative. I wasn't marrying into this family, so I spent the next four days partying. My uniform for the wedding was a large sombrero, orange snake-chaser-roach-killer-cowboy-boots, cut-off Levis, and the tuxedo coat, toting a five quart jug of that fine cactus juice we all call tequila—somehow I managed to screw up at the wedding anyway.

Larry had lost a bet to me in San Angelo. Payment was the orange cowboy boots. (For the uninformed, *snake-chasers* are the almost knee-high boots and *Roach-killers* are the really pointy boots. My attitude at that time was 'look good, feel good.') I tell you that was a very interesting four days. My wife has heard this story many times, so you can see why she might be concerned about my dressing.

Frustration

*P*art of my job now is to relieve my wife of as many duties as possible so she can perform as the breadwinner. I might also add she does this in a magnificent fashion. I can handle the housework all right, but there is no way I can work with money, so she still has to pay the bills and do all the things that have to do with money.

The complexity of frustration is interesting. It feeds on itself. When I do something that ends up in frustration, I have to be careful not to let that frustration carry over to the next thing I do. The more frustrated I get, the more frustrated I get. I think that makes sense. The frustration tends to make me blind to other situations. If I finish a project and end up frustrated from it, sometimes no matter how I try to fix my mind this plague carries over to my next job. Starting a task frustrated makes it that much easier to blow the next task. I find that most things I do aren't simple. I find catch-22s in just about everything I do. As an example, if I'm going to clean the house, I can't vacuum the carpet till I empty the vacuum bag. If I empty the vacuum bag I need to clean the vacuum at the same time.

To clean the carpet vacuum, I need to use the other vacuum that is the tile floor vacuum. As long as I'm going to have the tile vacuum out, should I do the tile floor first? Does the tile vacuum need to be emptied? If it does, what should I clean it with? Do I have clean bags for both vacuums? If I'm going to clean the tile vacuum with a spray cleaner, should I clean the tile first as long as I have the cleaner out? Well, you can see where I'm going with this. It is merely a matter of decision-making. Not a national problem of life and death, but to me this problem was enough for me to say to hell with it; I'll take a nap.

You may wonder, with that as my attitude, how the devil do I ever get anything done? At that point in my rehabilitation, I'm sure Denny wondered the same thing. Somehow or another, the cleaning seemed to always get done. Maybe not to her specs, but the big pieces were always picked up . . . mostly.

SOMETIMES IT JUST DOESN'T GO RIGHT

*D*enny was out of town and left me a passel of things to do. I've always been a list maker. Now I am a *plan maker* with a list. I can't make a plan if I don't have a list. This is a lesson in getting my plan and list to work together.

My wife has given me some things to do while she is away on business, as well as some things that need to be done around the house.

She left me a long list of everything so I wouldn't get lost, frustrated or flooded.

Several folks collect and save aluminum cans for me and the garage was in the process of being overrun with trash bags full of cans. So I'll start her list by cashing in cans. Drop Denny's boots at the shoe place. Be sure he puts taps on the toes—they are wearing out too fast—or does he have an alternative idea? Pick up the CDs from Diamond Records, be sure to order another Kingston Trio and a "Best of Johnny Horton." Ask John the owner if he found that song Denny hummed to him the last time we were in. Pick up the cleaning and be sure to check the stain that was on my peach-skin sport coat. It was on the right lapel. Stop at Walgreen's drugstore and pick up my Black Crow licorice. While I'm there look at Tums and if they are on sale buy three bottles. Otherwise we will get them Saturday. Go to Ace Hardware to pick up some Round Up. The architectural committee will site us if we don't do something about those weeds on the side of the house. While you're there, ask Bobby if he has anything cheaper that will do the job. Take a top back to Marshall's; it's too tight. Ask the sales gal if they have this same blouse in blue or green in a 34. When I'm finished with errands Denny wants me to get the van washed and gassed. She adds to that, "Don't forget to write down the trip mileage, the odometer reading and the date. Drop the convertible off at National and see if Bruce can fix the door locks."

She goes on to say, "Pill the pups; you have to stop at the vet's and get Shardak some *Rimadyl*. His hips are killing him, he can hardly get up. Your pills are in the skinny drawer. Don't take the ones in the small drawer. While you are at the vet's, get an appointment with Dr. Drow to get the cats their shots. Call the groomer's to see if they can takes Dancer Monday or Tuesday. I've got a presentation at Dell in Austin—if you want to make that trip with me that's great. If you can't go, you don't need to speak to the groomer about Dancer."

I'm already as busy as a one-legged man in a butt-kicking contest. On the way to cashing in the aluminum cans, a bag fell off the back of the convertible. It looked like someone had thrown a hand grenade comprised of coke cans. It took me twenty minutes to get that squared away. When I got to the recycling place, I found out Bob had put some non-aluminum in with the coke cans. By the look on the guy's face, you would have thought I had put a railroad track in there and was trying to rip him off. The shoe shop had a big sign saying he was out of business. John at the CD place wasn't able to get the CDs we wanted, maybe next week. The stain in my peach-skin sport coat was still there. Walgreen's was out of Black Crows. At Ace Hardware I paid top dollar for the weed killer. At Marshall's Department Store I couldn't get a sales girl to help me. Bruce said he didn't know what was wrong with the Caddy doors but if I left it there for a couple of days he would get it fixed for me. Sorry, but he had no idea what parts would cost, or even if he could get them. After all, Ruby is a 1984. When I got gas in Denny's van I wasn't paying attention and I put in the super-duper stuff for a super-duper price per gallon, rather than the lower octane, which it was supposed to have. I ended up spilling all my pills and couldn't remember which pills I took when. Hoorah, the vet worked out fine.

There was no way I was going to leave town, so I didn't have to worry about the dog groomer. All that folderol to tell you that even when you are prepared, things happen. Don't let them blow you away. None of this was life and death. When stuff like this happens, roll with it. Tomorrow will be a better day. Be prepared to have a plan "B" and "C". You never know when plan "A" is going to get blown away.

THOSE WHO STICK WITH YOU

I am fortunate with friends. I guess they chose well and so did I. Mentally-challenged folks have a rough time keeping good friends, that is BS to AS (Before Surgery to After Surgery).

Being cognitively-challenged is a non-communicable problem. You can't catch it by being in the same room with us or swapping body fluids. It is okay to hug; we will not bite your ears off. Shaking hands is allowed. Cheek kissing is allowed. If you have a mind to, it's okay to have sex.

Out of the clear blue I got a call from Goldie. I hadn't heard from him for twenty years, way BS (Before Surgery). I was very surprised, and very pleased because he has always been one of my favorite people. He was with me for a short time while I was getting my doctorate in survival. My wife and I went to his son's bar mitzvah. He showed me how to dress properly in a suit. Goldie arranged my one and only Mediterranean cruise as a sailor. He gave me a better handle on understanding humor. I wasn't about to forget who he was. We talked for quite some time reminiscing on our bumming from

Washington, DC to New Orleans for Mardi Gras where we stayed in a 'house of ill repute' and then were thrown in jail because we were mistaken for terrorists. This happened on the way to the West coast. On our trip from the West coast back to DC, we stopped in Wisconsin to visit my family. While we were there, we shoveled snow to pick up a couple of dollars to get us to DC. We shoveled snow for eight hours, then lost the money we made in a local poker game. We said enough of that, and pointed our thumbs back to DC to do some partying. I was working on my doctorate for survival, not common sense!

After hearing about my problem, Goldie still wanted to come visit. The visit was great; we learned what the other guy had been doing for the last twenty years or so. I was concerned about his wanting to be in touch after this visit, because I love the guy like a brother. He knows I'm different, but he says, "So what, so am I. We have both grown in twenty years. You just had some unusual circumstances put on you so you grew in a different way." Bless his heart! Goldie, always the diplomat. We still talk, and are making plans to get together again.

This same caring feeling I have goes to several old friends who have also been in touch. Ron, Larry, and Joe are others who helped me get my doctorate in survival, and many more guys and gals. I wish I could remember all the names, but you know, it's that old memory thing again. "God bless those who stick with us."

POOL

I have mentioned that my short- and long-term memory is impaired. Some of the things that I have forgotten are strange. For the last ten years I have played a pool game called nine ball most every Monday night with my friend Bob. When I was finally able to play again, Bob came over to the house. I was at the foot of the table getting ready to rack the balls, but I couldn't remember the positioning of the balls in the rack. Bob helped me. After a few games it hit me hard: I realized that my hand-eye coordination was not anywhere near as good as it used to be.

Before Surgery, Bob and I would split winning fifty/fifty. Now it was ninety/ten, Bob. He had to give me a tremendous handicap. That was very hard on my pool ego. At a time like that you find out who your *real* friends are. Most people would have just given up on me, but not Bob. He hung in there, reminded me of basic pool shots, gave me a few lessons and lots of encouragement. Never, never give up. It has taken two years to get back to the stage where we are more or less even again. Bob and I share a lottery number, I told him if we ever hit it,

I'll take up golf. Then he can spot me several shots and we can have another standing bet. That is if he can tolerate having two games to instruct me in. If there is something you want to do, hang in there. What you want may be like eating an elephant, but you can do it; just take one bite at a time.

POOL AND DARTS

Along the same lines as pool, I belonged to a dart league and found that I had forgotten some of the basics on how to play cricket. My teammates and the other teams we played were kind enough to help me along. One of the things that surprised me most was, when you're not playing darts, you should chalk (keep score for the people who are shooting). And, I couldn't keep track of the score; my math skills had failed me.

The games of 'three-o-one' and 'five-o-one' require simple math. I found that my math skills had deteriorated something fierce. My internal calculator was seriously broken. Subtracting a number like 39 from 301 seemed next to impossible. I just could not figure out how to do it. This added to my frustration, which in turn spilled over onto my dart throwing. Again I seemed to be in one of those circles like a catch-22. My chalking skills had to improve; hopefully this would help my dart throwing.

Fortunately, my dart buddies could see I was having a tough time of it. They would help with math and give me a beer break now and again to aid in frustration control. I must caution here, be careful about self-medication, dope, booze, etc. Too much of that stuff and you easily double the frustration factor. You have thrown in another variable and the more variables the harder something is to control. Remember this above all things: KISS—keep it simple stupid.

My wife was shopping one day and I was tagging along. I spotted this purse that had pockets and zippers all over it. I thought this purse will make a great dart bag. (I'm not one to worry about looking a little feminine.) I walked into Molly's one evening. (Molly's is the pub that sponsors our dart team.) One of the newer players was sitting having a beer. I sat down beside her, put my dart bag on the bar and Bonnie said, "Isn't that a purse?"

I said, "No, this is a dart bag. It was a purse in a former life but now it's a dart bag. Every now and again, particularly after I've had a beer or two, it reverts back to a purse, and every time it does I can never find my car keys."

Bonnie, being a purse carrier, said, "Yes, I know what you mean. I have the same problem if I have one too many beers."

We both laughed, and I said "As we sit here talking, this is a dart bag, but who knows what it will be a couple of hours from now."

My wrist was bothering me so I had stopped and got a wrist brace on my way to darts. When I walked into Molly's, Ann, one of my old teammates, stopped me and asked, "What did you do to your wrist?"

I enjoy playing with people's minds now and again, and besides Ann is an old, dear friend with a great sense of humor. So I told her, "Oh didn't you hear? My teammates got together and approached Lloyd's of London to have my arm insured for a million dollars. Lloyd's said yes, but if I am *not* shooting, I have to wear a protective arm brace."

She said, "No kidding?"

I said, "Ann, who is the brain-damaged one here, you or me?" She laughed and walked away. Bless her heart, she may not have thought it was funny but she saw that I thought it was, and went along with it. The whole dart league laughs *with me* instead of at me. We all need this kind of support, brain-damaged or not.

FLEXIBILITY, PANIC, COMMUNICATIONS

A simple task and plan is materializing: Denny's van was in the shop. I was going to give her a ride up to Conroe, a small town thirty or so miles away. (She's found that a small town is better for negotiating, so she bought her last two vans there.) We will pick up her van and I will follow her back to the house. We'll drop off my convertible, then I will take over driving the van to run errands, then we will go to lunch. We both carry cell phones. We picked up the car and I began following my wife; all is well.

She changed lanes, and increased her speed and I lost sight of her. Our turn was coming up. I saw a break in the traffic and put my foot on it so I could catch up with her. Just as I caught up I saw her going past our turn. The adrenaline shot up to my bald spot. This was not in the plan. What had happened? I called her on the cell phone and asked, "What is going on?"

She said, "Sorry I forgot to tell you, I need gas."

Later I told her how badly the adrenaline hit me when I saw her pass our usual turn. From that point on, if our plans change, I get a phone call first. If you have a problem like mine, get a cell phone. The peace of mind and feeling of security are well worth the small expense. A cell phone alleviates a lot of flooding. No matter how bad things get, I know my wife is just a phone call away. That's very comforting. When I forget the phone, I feel like Linus when Lucy and Snoopy have done something with his blanket. Yes, the cell phone is a security blanket for me, and I love it.

Any variations to a plan tax the inflexible part of my brain to its limits. As I told my wife, "Let's not push any limits of my deficit areas unless we preplan it. Day-to-day living tends to bring me enough surprises."

It is good to test limits, and grow the weak areas; that's one way of getting new synapses snapping. But keep in mind it is hard to learn when you are flooding. So grow the deficit areas intelligently. Plan ahead, when possible. Make sure you challenge yourself every day. Make your comfort zone bigger with each challenge. As you are creating the new you, make sure you create a person you would be proud to be friends with, not a scaredy-cat with tunnel vision.

POKER

My wife and I were grocery shopping and we ran into Teddy, an old friend and poker buddy. I hadn't seen him since BS (Before Surgery). He told me about a small poker game he played in and asked if I would be interested. I had thought about playing poker several times and even though there was a time when I made my living playing a reasonably high stakes game, I was now fearful of getting into a game.

This game was effectively a penny ante game. Well, close to it: it was a dollar limit. Denny spoke with my counselors and decided that any money I might lose would be well worth the therapy I would get out of using my executive functioning skills (what little I had left).

The game started promptly at 7:00 p.m. and the last deal was at eleven. No wild cards period, although they do play some off-the-wall games. When I was introduced to the game on the first night, Steve said, "We've got wild games and wild players, but no wild cards."

How about this for strange? You start out with a Ruffus deal. What's a Ruffus deal, you say? Randy played with a friend when he was a kid who dealt all the down cards at one time. So if you're playing draw poker you get the next five cards, the next guy gets the next five cards and so on. So if you're playing Stewy—What's a Stewy? Four cards down, to each player (of course, that's a Ruffus deal). Five cards down in the middle of the table. These are common cards that the dealer turns over. When the dealer turns the third card, it's a Stewy. Seven or below in that suit or eight and above in the hole wins half the pot.

That's not near our strangest game. It would take too long to go into the details of the more interesting games. We play another game the players call Cross-Dresser. You might know it as Utah. But the players say if you play that game you always carry a matching purse, and underwear. Teddy, who was one of the charter members of this poker club, is very good at playing the Cross-Dresser game. I'm sure he plays this game to blow the other players' minds.

One Wednesday evening, it was Teddy's deal. He said, "We're playing Cross-Dresser."

Mike looked at him and said, "Teddy, are you wearing a tutu again? You always play that sissy game!"

Teddy pulled Mike's leg a little further and said, "Teddy is wearing a teddy."

This gave us all a laugh.

Steve interjected, "To think I tell people we don't play any sissy-girl games in this here poker parlor. What a joke that is."

Keep in mind, these guys are men's men. Any one of them is capable of tearing off somebody's head just so they could yell down their neck to see if there's an echo. For the most part they are all sweethearts.

I still remembered which hand beats what, but I couldn't remember any of the strategies involved. I remember my first game at Steve's Rock Yard & Poker Parlor. This is a cement block building in the middle of a stone yard. Steve is a man who builds waterfalls and such. He is a big man with a commanding personality. It wouldn't surprise me at all if one of his customers were to ask for a replica of Niagara Falls in their back yard for him to say, "Certainly, but it'll cost you extra for diverting the Rio Grande."

I told the players to keep an eye on me, that if I made a mistake, it's not because I'm a cheater. I told them I was brain-damaged and if I didn't work out, I would walk away with no bad feelings. It was very uncomfortable for all of us at first. They weren't sure just what *brain-damaged* meant. Was I crazy, stupid, or what? Today there is no problem; they treat me just like the other guys who play—brain-damaged. Now and then I wonder about some of these guys. Some of the hands they stay in on are hard to believe, but then I do it myself, too. I tell them if I were good at this, I would make my living at it.

One evening I beat Randy out of a hand. I dealt the next hand, and gave Randy a second best.

He says, "That's it Dick, I'm putting the juju on you."

Juju is a bad luck curse. It comes from Africa and the Caribbean and it made me think about the people I go to rehab with. Somebody or some thing has put the juju on them. Randy would pass the juju on to anybody who beat him several times in a row.

All in all, these guys are a bunch of decent poker players. They are good men who care about each other and through the last couple of years I've watched them help each other out of tight spots, loan money, win alot, and lose alot. The friendships stay strong. I wish the rest of the world were like these guys—no pretense: what you see is what you get, and if you don't like it, tough shit. Get out.

I never realized how much of my executive functioning skills were involved in playing poker. I have to decide what to deal, get some kind of a plan, remember all the cards that were played as well as the cards that are up. Calculate my odds on the strategy that I have chosen as the cards are dealt and be prepared to change strategy. My old nemesis, *cognitive inflexibility* would get a good workout at these games. Be observant of who is betting, how and why. Make a judgment call on every card as to whether I want to call, raise or get out. Of course, the final and biggest judgment was, "Can my hand beat every other hand at the table, or do I have a hand that I could consider trying a bluff?" Bluffing is a few and far between event, because you can't get these guys out with dynamite. That's part of the fun. I have to learn to use that as a ploy.

On occasion we will play a game called *low Chicago*. This is a seven card stud game with the low spade in the hole getting half the pot and the best poker hand getting the other half. I have at one time or another come to the seventh card and discovered I had no poker hand and dropped out, later thinking to myself that I had the deuce of spades in the hole. That means I just threw away half that pot. Well, if I were good at this game I'd make my living at it.

These guys are great! They all know I'm brain-damaged and they help me out. One time when I was actually dealing backwards, one of the guys said, "Dick, you're dealing backwards."

I kept dealing and said, "Does anyone care?" Bless their hearts, they couldn't care less. Dino said, "After all, how bad can it be if we allow a Ruffus deal?"

Poker does more than just work on my weak cognitive areas. There was a time when I hadn't laughed for two years (the snuggie suit era), so this next piece of info says magnitudes about the value of these guys and this game to me.

One night Scott came in after we had started. While he was getting organized with his buy-in, he was telling us jokes. The man knows how to tell a joke, and he had six of us in belly laughs for several minutes. It had been a long time since I laughed so hard that my facial muscles were sore and my sides ached. We all laughed and carried on. It was great. I'm happy to say that Scott gave us many, many of these. The only thing better for releasing tension, anxiety, frustration and all those other bad guys would be to have a knocked-out love session with my wife. Everyone needs both kinds of outlets. If Scott could figure out how to bottle that stuff, it would be the greatest antidepressant ever. Goodbye Prozac.

Scott is a guy who has had some bad times over the last year or so. Along with his personal problems, I think Randy's juju must have escaped its usual resting place and bitten poor old Scott right on the butt. He has been drawing garbage or second best hand for the last couple of months. I must say, he is a game dude. We see him every other week or so. He is testing the waters to see if the juju has lit on anyone else. The man has got stick-to-itiveness. I admire his ability to get us all belly laughing when his own life is not all cherries.

Sure enough, Randy's juju jumped on someone else. Scott hasn't changed a dram. When he comes to a game, the rest of us plan on going home with sore facial muscles and sore stomach muscles and a lot less anxiety, frustration and tension.

Something I learned from Scott as well as my fellow rehabbers is "Get back up on the horse." If you don't quit, you don't lose. I wonder if Scott needs or would like to join our rehab group. I think he is more crazy than brain-damaged.

Brain Damage

My affirmation from this poker game is "I look for humor in as many things as I can. I will learn from my mistakes and repeat them as little as possible." I'm working on my vocabulary, retention and retrieval with this affirmation in mind. I explained the poker game with some details to show you I am going to learn from every experience I can. I did learn a little something from one of the guys, Randy (the Champion Coral Snake Wrestler)—not to be confused with "Ju-Ju Randy." The coral snake wrestler is not a herpetologist either, as you will see. Randy, the coral snake wrestler, had consumed one beer too many at home. His wife told him there was a snake on the porch, and would he please get rid of it. He thought it was a king snake; when he picked it up, the snake bit him twice. He is the only man I have ever heard of who was bitten by a coral snake *twice* and lived to tell about it. The lesson I have learned from this is that all guns are loaded and all snakes are poisonous. When you are handling snakes or guns, this is a good thing to keep in mind. (I just threw in the part about guns, cause it seems to fall into the same category as poisonous snakes, safety-wise, that is.)

I am pleased to add that I give Denny a percentage of my winnings. I list this under poker because that is where I win the most money. Every now and again I get lucky at darts. If the league is having a blind draw contest and if I draw one of the top flight dart shooters and if I'm on at all, I stand a chance of picking up a couple of bucks. At any rate, my wife gets a couple of dollars if I do. She calls it *mad money.* She can blow this on whatever she wants and it doesn't affect the household budget. She may buy a pair of earrings or a blouse. No matter how you cut it, it makes me feel good, almost like I'm a contributor.

PARTY BRIDGE

*B*ridge to me is the card player's chess game. All the games I play interact with each other. Card games help me improve my executive functioning skills. My bridge-playing and poker-playing help improve each other. The darts and pool playing help improve my hand-eye coordination. I'm fortunate to be married to someone who understands their value.

Some less caring person might say, "Yea, yea, that's just a couple of nights out with the boys." I thank all the powers that be for the woman I have.

I had known the bridge players for a number of years BS (Before Surgery). They tell me they can't see much difference in my playing BS or AS (After Surgery). What does that say about my level of bridge playing? I had to go back to the basics for bridge. For instance the finesse was a strange play for me. I couldn't understand why I should play my queen to my ace. It seemed dumb to put my ace on my queen (not thinking that if the king didn't show up, I didn't have to do that).

Pre-empts were also strange. Why do I need points when I have all that trump?

Eventually, I remembered the basics. Retaining the rules, etiquette, bids and responses from one game to the next is still challenging. I don't play in Omar Sharif's class, but I don't embarrass myself much, too often.

SUPPER CLUB

For twenty years, we have belonged to a supper club in our subdivision. There are ten couples. We have been fortunate enough to keep the original group, with some fine exceptions, Bill and Mary-Jo.

For twenty years it has been a standing joke that to be invited to be a member for the next year you must have committed some type of social *faux pas* at supper club the year before. A couple of the social errors stick in my mind. One of my favorites was committed early, just after the forming of our group. After a rather long cocktail period we sat down for soup. A gal sitting at our table made the comment that she thought another woman's hair looked exceptionally nice. The woman thanked her and we went on with the conversation. The first woman cut into the conversation several more times to say again how nice her hair looked. After the third interruption I could see everyone at our table was getting slightly miffed at this one-track interruption. Upon the fourth interruption I heard, "Apparently you really like this hairdo." She took off her wig and threw it at the woman and said, "Here, you can have it."

Of course the wig landed in the soup. At first everybody was appalled at the way the problem was handled. The other lady carefully, with two fingers, picked this dead rat-looking thing out of her soup and put it on the floor. The whole place was quiet for a moment and then burst out in uproarious laughter. Shortly after that, several toasts to the dead rat and, between courses, the guy across from me made me a substantial bet that I couldn't do ten chin-ups. We happened to be in a modern home with exposed beams. I promptly stood on my chair, stepped on the table and gave him ten chin-ups from the exposed beam. Well, this was to set a precedent for the *faux pas* thing.

Later, the other supper club members told me that this *faux pas* would give me life-long membership in the supper club. Since then, we have had such minor social errors as chili and red wine spilled on brand new white wall-to-wall carpet, or diving into a swimming pool and losing the top or bottom of your suit, or falling into the hot tub fully clothed. These didn't seem as colorful as the drowned rat happening, but they were good enough to get the perpetrators invited to be in next year's supper club.

Ed is a member in high standing in the bridge group and the supper club. He prides himself in his loud shirt collection. He should; his collection is the envy of anybody who has ever wanted a so-called Hawaiian shirt. When it comes to wild shirts, Ed is in a class by himself. I have never been one to desire loud shirts. Denny has bought a lot of shirts for me because of my reluctance to buy new stuff. She has bought me a couple of outstanding loud shirts and I am now enjoying purple palm trees, orange birds, mauve pineapples and the like. We like to call them *sayin-sumthin'* shirts. This loud shirt thing is new for me, After Surgery. It's a different and fun thing and I'm enjoying it. I'm trying to move into Ed's class, but I fear I have a long way to go. My wife says, "Hang in there, Dick. We'll shop every beach store in the Caribbean till we find one or two that will put a smile on the face of that owner of the wildest shirt collection in Texas, Ed."

I told her that is a very ambitious goal, but then again I like the challenge of an ambitious goal. Plus we can check out beaches, piña coladas and local breweries in the process. See there, ambition and goals give a person all kinds of rewards.

SILLINESS

My wife was telling this story at supper club and I happened to have overheard it. She was at an airport helping a fellow salesperson. The teammate was aware of my situation. They were rushing to catch a plane which always seems to be the case when Denny is at an airport.

The friend said, "What gate are we looking for?"

My wife replied, "I forgot, because my husband is brain damaged."

The teammate said, "You can't use that as an excuse."

Denny said, "Why not? My husband uses it all the time."

This brought a chuckle or two from the listeners. I stepped into the conversation and said, "Well that sure is a new slant on 'I was having a senior moment.' You might just as well tell these people the last time we made love you caught my brain damage. We could start a whole new thing about sexually transmitted poor memory." You can't catch poor memory like that, can you?

Denny and I were in a restaurant. I was looking around to see who else was in the room.

She reached across the table and touched my arm. Then said, "You didn't hear what I said, did you?"

"No, I was giving the place the once over, to see who's here."

She said, "Your hearing seems to be challenged. Did they, by any chance, break your listener when they broke your memory?"

I said, "Eh? What's that you say?"

As a brain-damaged guy, and the wife of a brain-damaged guy, we try to find humor whenever and wherever we can.

Cry in your beer or try and find the light side. Look for stuff to kid each other about.

THE UPSIDE TO BEING BRAIN-DAMAGED

I had commented to my wife that there are some good aspects to being brain-damaged. I am a *Star Trek* fan and when the reruns came back on it was great: I remembered that I had seen this episode, but I couldn't remember what happened next. I get to see all my old favorite movies almost as new. My wife's comment was taken directly from the book *Over My Head*.

She said "Yes, and now you can hide your own Easter eggs."

Part of my rehabilitation is that I create the new Dick. This one will be wise, eager to learn, tender, a good lover, sensitive, a good listener, a good friend and conscientious about improving all facets of my relationships and myself. I will be a writer. I will help people (who are brain-damaged) through my stories. I will help kids (who have lost hope) with my fantasy books. I will help people who want to get an education to get one. I will be more thankful for the things I have and to the folks who have helped me. This is not a New Year's resolution; this is my new way of life.

It is amazing what I had to go through to detect flaws in my character. I am in charge of who I am and what I am. Something just happened and I have control. As an example, I am dyslexic.

I found out well into adulthood that I suffered from dyslexia. (No wonder I failed two years of history.) I also found that doing crossword puzzles seemed to help with this. Now, for some unknown reason (since the brain surgery), my dyslexic problem has improved. I don't skip letters nearly as often when I am writing or doing crosswords. I wonder how many other improvements I will find through the years. You can bet your best boots I'll be looking for them.

I'm still very much alive, so I'm still developing the new me. As far as I'm concerned I will be developing the new me till I cross over, and who knows what then?

EMOTIONS RUN WILD

I started crying a lot, even during *TV* commercials. It doesn't take a genius to figure it out: you can bet your best hound dog that if you see someone crying over a commercial, chances are pretty good that person has a broken emotional control switch.

Welcome to the wonderful world of brain-damage. When this starts, I can feel the emotions pulling on me like someone twanging a 1,000 pound bowstring. My eyes start to fill with water and my gut gets tight. I don't mind tearing up for a good reason—*Old Yeller, Bryan's Song,* or something like that. Reminds me of a quote from Henry Fonda. Someone asked him if he was an emotional man and he said, "I'll cry over a good steak." It's like someone else is in charge and hits this emotion button for no reason. Unfortunately, this type of crying is not an emotional release. It is frustrating, and I am unable to figure out why I do this, which in turn, adds to the frustration. Until you play in this ballpark, cut some slack for those of us who do.

I am told by those folks who know that I will probably have a broken emotional switch forever. So be it. I'll learn to live with it.

INTERNAL THERMOSTAT

Having no pituitary gland (or a non-functional pituitary) has lots of side affects. One of them is that my internal temperature control does not work worth a darn. This makes for some curious events.

Most people have internal thermostats that work pretty much the same, for example if you're out in the hot Texas sun, you're hot. Then when you go into a restaurant, the temperature is cool inside, and in a few moments, you probably feel comfortable.

With me, if I go from hot outside to cool inside, I freeze to death. It's like falling into an icy river. In other cases, while somebody may feel warm in a room, I will be roasting, like having a dragon breathe fire on me. I wonder how the dragon likes his meat cooked and when he is going to turn the spit.

One of the worst things about having a broken thermostat has to do with intimacy. I remember when my wife and I first got married, part of the excitement was the touching of the bodies. Now, I have to wear socks and a T-shirt or I freeze to death. I told my wife, "All I have to do is get one of those

Groucho Marx glasses and nose, then we can make our own fifties stag films."

Thank goodness she sees the humor in this and is willing to put up with me.

TO YOU, FOR YOU, THE READER

*T*he Center for Disease Control has said "Each year 260,000 people are hospitalized with traumatic brain injury."

There are a lot of folks to help and that doesn't count the friends and relatives of those disabled people. You could easily say that well over a million people a year are affected by cognitive-impairment in one way or another.

Someone in your life has helped you. Pass it on. Now, you have helped somebody. Wars start with a single action. Why not peace? Who knows, maybe we can start a tsunami of peace and love. We damn sure won't if we don't try.

We all need more *pleases* and *thank yous*, more smiles, more *I cans* and fewer *no I can'ts*. Don't be a person who wears blinders or has tunnel-vision. Be open-minded; look for new and different ideas. You don't have to try them all, but you should at least know there are options out there for most everything. Look for what is important to you as far as quality of life is concerned. Then go for it! If you know someone else needs more quality of life, and you can help, do it! Be mentally active, grow your comfort zone. Do new things, learn something new every day, even if it is only a new word.

Sounds like life, doesn't it? Make the best decisions you can, then learn by the good choices as well as the bad ones.

If you want to know how to help someone else, find a rehabilitation center. Here, Project ReEntry has questionnaires that help determine your area of interest. This is not a pass/fail type of test; it is designed to eliminate things you don't want to do, then point you in a new direction.

I give you this from Paul J. Meyer. It is a master plan for being successful. You complete it by deciding what success means to you:

> *"Whatever you vividly imagine,*
> *Ardently desire,*
> *Sincerely believe,*
> *And enthusiastically act upon...*
> *Must inevitably come to pass!"*

I leave you with my wife's favorite poem (author unknown):

> *I have a premonition*
> *It soars on silver wings.*
> *I dream of your accomplishments*
> *and other wondrous things.*
> *I do not know beneath which sky*
> *Nor where you'll challenge fate.*
> *I only know it will be high.*
> *I only know you will be great!*

Afterword from his Counselor

An enduring memory of Richard "Dick" Schmelzkopf is burned into my brain. Many summer days when he would leave our brain injury treatment facility, Project ReEntry, he would get into his maroon convertible automobile, which he calls "Ruby." With the top down he would take off his shirt, put on his sunglasses, light up one of those skinny little ginseng cigarettes and head out for parts unknown with his thinning hair blowing in the wind. This memory epitomizes the man for me. He does things his way. No matter how strange it may seem to others. I don't believe his brain injury had anything to do with this wonderfully quirky side of his personality.

I direct the outpatient brain injury treatment programs at Project ReEntry. I was also the first therapist to work with Mr. Schmelzkopf when he began our program. He is one of the most world-wise people I know. Even from the first day of treatment in Project ReEntry, he entertained all that would listen with colorful jokes and his experiences in the Navy. At first, the jokes were too colorful and he had to be reminded that there was a time and a place for those kinds of jokes and this was neither. As always, he took the feedback about his behavior well. OK, the truth is, early on in our rehabilitation efforts with him he was not as open to feedback as he is now. In fact, he could not fathom that he could be wrong about anything. This is a familiar reaction by clients who suffer from closed head injuries. Even though he does not suffer from a closed head injury, he experiences many of the same cognitive impairments, or thinking problems, as do closed head injury clients.

Mr. Schmelzkopf had a brain tumor removed from the pituitary region of his brain on June 2, 1994. He participated in a neuropsychological battery of tests with our practice, Larry Pollock, Ph.D., and Associates, on January 8, 1996. His reported disability of a Brain Tumor was accompanied by his subjective complaints of forgetting, of reduced ability to plan and organize information, and of difficulty following conversations. It was noted in the neuropsychological evaluation that he related stories of forgetting to turn off the stove, forgetting to shut the refrigerator door and forgetting to unload the dishwasher. He also lamented that he forgot how to operate a computer even though that was a significant part of his previous employment as a regional sales manager. The results of the neuropsychological evaluation revealed a diagnosis of Organic Brain Injury and Depressive Disorder. Organic Brain Syndrome is a constellation of cognitive deficits that describes impairments in brain functioning.

My first opportunity to meet Mr. Schmelzkopf was during the Specialized Brain Injury Functional Evaluation that he participated in on January 31, 1996. He stated that his vocational goal was to return to sales and he also wanted to write children's stories. My next encounter with him was during the meeting where we reviewed all the results of the evaluations he underwent with our practice. At this meeting I had the opportunity to meet his wife, Denise. An angel if there ever was one. She has the patience of Job and the strength of character to help Dick through his ordeal. She would not give up on Dick or allow him to give up on himself. I truly believe he would not be where he is today without her. We recommended him for our treatment program at this meeting. He began treatment with Project ReEntry on July 9, 1996.

Treatment began normally enough with Mr. Schmelzkopf. He was given a treatment plan to address the cognitive deficits that were identified during his neuropsychological evaluation. He politely agreed that he needed to work on them and then proceeded to do things his way. Our big push in the treatment program is for clients with memory problems to take notes and refer back to them often. In the beginning, he saw no reason to take down notes on "every little thing." Because of this lack of note taking, he was often late to group therapies that he did not write down on his schedule. He also could not remember instructions on tasks therapists gave him. The more we insisted that he take notes, the more he resisted. So we stopped insisting. Rather, we let him structure his own treatment. This was great news to him.

It was at this time, in November of 1996, that we began working with Mr. Schmelzkopf almost exclusively on his writing projects. Many of the therapeutic interventions with him focused on vocabulary building and other language-related tasks. It was also our intentions to help him to plan and organize more efficiently. To that end I helped him set up an outline to work on his lifelong passion, a children's book. He had no idea how to go about setting up an outline for such a task. I had no doubt that this was due to the damage caused by the brain tumor. He functioned in a high-level capacity in his previous work and most certainly would have been able to do something as simple as outlining a project. I remember sitting and discussing with him what he wanted to do with this book, what the characters would do, where it would take place, how the chronology would run and many other details. We began the outline in the word processor using the Microsoft Word program. He was very excited. The very next treatment session started with him huffing and puffing into my office and exclaiming that he lost all of the work we had done previously. He saw no need to write down the instructions I had given him regarding the operation of the computer and he could not start the program nor could he open the file. Knowing the importance of this project to him, I had saved this file to our computer's hard drive before he had left on the previous treatment session. It was then that he saw the value in taking notes and referring to them often. This was an epiphany for him in dealing with his disability. He now realized how his memory problems and his difficulties with planning and organization could impact his future goals.

At this same time, in the fall of 1996, Mr. Schmelzkopf signed up for a writing course at a local college. He wanted to start learning the craft he someday hoped would lead to publishing his first children's book. He subsequently got involved with a writers' group that critiqued each other's work as a result of his contacts with the college. This is where he met his "guru." I only know her name as Guida and she became his literary guiding light. She gave him the technical side of writing that he needed at that time. He became very focused on his writing during this time. He and his wife both commented that he was thinking more clearly and able to accept feedback more readily than in previous months. The cognitive rehabilitation and the writing classes were a perfect antidote for what ailed him at the time.

The first creative success for Mr. Schmelzkopf came at Project ReEntry. We were having an appreciation luncheon for several referral sources during the month of May 1997. We were going to make a video tape of clients in therapy to show "a typical day" at Project ReEntry. He offered to script the whole tape with him doing the "voice-over" describing what cognitive therapy is and how clients benefit from it from a client's perspective. He worked for days on the text of the speech. He consulted with the Project ReEntry staff as well as with other participants in our treatment program, He really wanted this project to be a meaningful and truthful expression of what cognitive therapy means from a client's perspective. The video could not be shown because one of the clients withdrew permission to show it at the last minute. However, we did play his audio tape explaining the brain injury rehabilitation process. There were about 50 people in attendance, excluding our staff, and he received a standing ovation. He beamed from ear to ear. He so enjoyed the recognition of his efforts that it was right then and there that I believe he decided to write his own rehabilitation story.

The ensuing months saw Mr. Schmelzkopf working hard on his children's book that we all referred to as "Purpose." As the book grew ever larger as he added chapter after chapter, we realized that he was not able to organize his story line very well.

He was also making numerous grammatical errors in his writing.

In September of 1998, Dr. Pollock agreed to take on the challenge of helping Dick pull Purpose all together. He began meeting weekly with Dick to address these issues. Dick was initially a little defensive about making changes to "his" story but he eventually saw the benefit in what Dr. Pollock was teaching him. He began to see all of the verb tense shifting and how the chronology of the story line had problems. He began making corrections and checking them with Dr. Pollock and with his guru.

About the beginning of 1999, he began trying to market interest in his book project. We worked with him on all the resources we could identify that might help him. He began sending out letters to publishers with no luck. He became frustrated with the scope of the task of finishing this book. The book was approaching a novel in length. He was tiring of the numerous corrections he was having to make constantly. His interest starting waning and he began thinking about other projects, much to our chagrin. We wanted him to focus on one thing at a time and see it through. But he has his own way of doing things and started on a couple of other projects around the end of 1999.

Mr. Schmelzkopf very much enjoys the sport of Darts. He wrote a story about darts that he referred to as the "Darty Story" that was published on a web page of a local restaurant and bar establishment. He was encouraged again.

Mr. Schmelzkopf then began writing his personal rehabilitation story in earnest at the end of 1999. We agreed to help him go forward with this project. He began much the same as when he first started in treatment with our program, except that he

Afterword from his Counselor

was doing all the outlining this time. He had some rough spots but he was able to organize his thoughts more efficiently on this project than with the first one. It was heart-warming to say the least. It's exactly what therapists want for their clients. He was independently using all of the cognitive compensatory strategies that we had been preaching for three years. He worked tirelessly on his story. He accepted input from his guru, from the Project ReEntry treatment team and from his wife. Before I knew it, he was coming in saying that someone from Emerald Ink Publishing was interested in his story and wanted to see the first three chapters of his story. For the first time, I could see confidence welling up inside him. Someone had just given credence to the last four years of his life. Maybe he could make a future out of writing. He is back in the driver's seat again.

Russell Shanks, M.A.
Director of Project ReEntry

From the Director of the Facility

*D*uring the past 25 years, I have had the privilege of evaluating and treating thousands of patients who have suffered brain injury from a wide variety of causes. Each one of these survivors has a unique story, and each has struggled with their own special set of challenges and opportunities. However, there are many common themes which these survivors and their families discover as they go through the process of creating a new person. Although most hospitals and rehabilitation centers provide educational material for brain injury survivors and their families, no amount of professional jargon or medical information can adequately communicate the adventure which lies ahead for every survivor. In fact, my experience has shown that other survivors and their families are the best source of information for people who have recently suffered a brain injury. In fact, support groups such as those sponsored by the National

Brain Injury Association and by many rehabilitation centers are one of the best mechanisms for preparing "new rehabbers" for the ups and downs which are an inevitable part of the recovery process. I have participated in many of these groups over the years and have witnessed incredible warmth and empathy which the a relatively small number of brain injury survivors. Many survivors do not have an opportunity to participate in such a group and miss out on the many benefits which they provide. Consequently, they do not have an opportunity to share their experiences with others who have already been through the process. As a result, they often feel alone and isolated. There is also a lack of support groups for the families of brain injury survivors. Thus, many family members have difficulty understanding what their loved one is going through and are often confused and upset by the "new person" who is emerging as a result of the rehabilitation process.

Fortunately, when Dick Schmelzkopf entered Project ReEntry, he and his wife, Denny, had already done substantial research and were already making some excellent adjustments to Dick's brain injury. Nevertheless, they still had many doubts and questions which they eagerly explored with the other "rehabbers" at Project ReEntry and with our staff. Dick quickly became an outspoken leader among the patients and was a very active participant in all of our treatment groups. Whether the topic of the group was stress management, self-esteem, or men's issues, he always brought an interesting combination of thoughtfulness, creativity and humor to the discussions. As his own insights and awareness evolved, he became an important source of empathy and support for the other participants. Dick's care and concern for the well-being of his fellow rehabbers has been one of his outstanding qualities during his participation at Project ReEntry. Consequently, I was not surprised when he approached me about his desire to write a book about "life after brain injury." His goal was to provide helpful insights and information for patients who had recently suffered a brain injury and who were still trying to figure out what had happened to them and what they were going through. I encouraged Dick to pursue this idea because there is definitely a void in this area of educational literature. Although there are a few books and articles on this topic, brain injury survivors and their families usually have difficulty finding material which helps them relate to the changes in their life and the new experiences which they are encountering. And, as a therapist, I felt that it would be a wonderful cognitive rehabilitation activity that would assist with Dick's recovery!

Writing this book did prove to be an excellent rehabilitation project for Dick. From a cognitive perspective, it was another exercise in which he was able to practice and hone his planning and organizational skills. Dick had many great ideas for the book but for a while he had difficulty initiating and following through on them. For quite a while, he was preoccupied with jotting down humorous anecdotes and other topics that he wanted to include in the book. During this period, he made limited progress toward writing the book. In order to overcome this obstacle, Dick worked closely with our clinical psychologist, Dr. Marta Rosenberg, to develop timely outlines and a schedule

From the Director of the Facility

for converting his many ideas into a written transcript. The act of converting his thoughts and ideas into written paragraphs was another major therapeutic activity on which this book enabled him to work. After his brain injury, Dick found it difficult to put his wonderful, creative thoughts into writing. Our treatment team spent many hours helping him find strategies that would help him express his creative ideas in a writing style that would reflect his articulate and humorous style of speech.

I have been involved with various aspects of rehabilitation for over 30 years. During that time I have been asked on successful rehab program, but I am personally convinced that successful rehabilitation depends on the "indomitable human spirit." When patients have an intense desire to achieve their goals, they often accomplish things that no one could ever predict. Dick Schmelzkopf is an inspiring example of what that "indomitable human spirit" can achieve. When he entered Project ReEntry, no one but Dick would ever have dreamed that he could complete two major books within a two and a half year period of time. And, if I know Dick, "You ain't seen nothin' yet!"

Larry Pollock, Ph.D.
Clinical Neuropsychologist
Executive Director of Project ReEntry

OTHER TITLES BY EMERALD INK

Business & Home
Debt Control, Chris Richards, ISBN 1-885373-19-8
Start A Business Without Borrowing, D. Kelly Irvin, ISBN 1-885373-05-8
The Art of Persuasion, Forrest Watson, Ph.D., ISBN 1-885373-46-5
The Network Marketer, Forrest Watson, Ph.D., ISBN 1-885373-37-6
Understanding & Reducing Your Home Electric Bill, Richard L. Hepburn, MS, ISBN 1-885373-01-5

Fiction
Colorado Bound, Eddie Dean Trammell, ISBN 1-885373-45-7
Offahore, Don Corace, ISBN 0-9760426-0-6
The Pokhraj, Irina Gajjar, ISBN 1-885373-44-9

Health/Mental Health
Brain Damage, Dick Schmelzkopf, ISBN 1-885373-34-1
Conquering Kid's Cancer, Ken Lazaraus, MD, ISBN 1-885373-22-8
How I Conquered Cancer (naturopathic prostate), Eric Gardiner, ISBN 1-885373-11-2 How To Survive Your Bipolar Brain, Bob Bradley, ISBN 1-885373-43-0
Manic Depression: How To Live While Loving a Manic Depressive, Lynn Bradley, ISBN 1-885373-28-7
Sexual Health, Doris Zale, RN, ISBN 1-885373-26-0

History/Memoirs/Travel/Ghosts
The Black Walnut Farm, Ted Woodworth, ISBN 1-885373-52-X
Childhood Memories of the Great Depression, Ted Woodworth, ISBN 1-885373-29-5
From China With Love, Lou Glist, ISBN 1-885373-60-0
Growin' Up Poor, Ted Woodworth, ISBN 1-885373-53-8 *Rebel Private*, Wm. A. Fletcher, ISBN 1-885373-42-2
Reflections of A Rotarian, Jack Pearce, ISBN 1-885373-03-1
Spirits of Texas (true Texas ghosts), Vallie Fletcher Taylor, ISBN 1-885373-40-6
The Celestial Kingdom, Stephen Andree, ISBN 1-885373-5-2

Mystery
Set Sail for Murder, Lynn Bradley, ISBN 1-885373-47-3

Social
It's U-Mail! Lighthearted Guide to Enhancing Intuition, Robert Stecker, Ph.D., ISBN 1-885373-20-1
Love Now, Here's How (removing roadblocks to relationships), Phyllis Light, Ph.D., ISBN 1-885373-36-8
Prince Charming Lives, Phyllis Light, Ph.D., ISBN 1-885373-38-4
Society & Sex Offenders, Ray Mullen, MSW, ISBN 1-885373-14-7

Spiritual
Crossing Over & Coming Home (gay/lesbian NDEs), Liz Dale, Ph.D., 1-885373-32-5
Mary of Galilee (narrative of early life of Mary), Frances Woodard, ISBN 1-885373-23-6
Memory of Elsewhere (reflections on meaning), Rona Murray Dexter, Ph.D., ISBN 1-885373-35-X
Return From the Sunset, Richard Trask, ISBN 1-885373-33-3
The Spiritual Dimension of the Gay & Lesbian Experience, Daniel Helminiak, ISBN 1-885373-59-7
When Ego Dies—A Compilation of Near-Death & Mystical Conversion Stories, ISBN 1-885373-07-4
You Know Me—The Gita (Bhagavad Gita), tr. Irina Gajjar, Ph.D., ISBN 1-885373-27-9

True Crime
Undercover Knights, Ben Lucas, ISBN 1-885373-39-2